AF679398

Mysteries
Of The
Mitochondria

Charles R Giardina

Copyright © 2025 Charles R Giardina. All rights reserved for data mining, text, A.I. technologies and similar training.

Mysteries
Of The
Mitochondria

Unveiling Quantum and Cancer

A treatise, based on the thesis that cancer is a metabolic disease. With an in-depth descriptions of:

- Basics of Mitochondria
- Quantum Tunneling
- Mitochondria Dysfunction And Cancer

The fundamental message of the text is that cancer should be acknowledged to be a metabolic disease. Remission could be around the corner with proper life style and diet. Numerous descriptions as well as over a hundred references are provided, illustrating why this is possible. In particular, Dr. Seyfried's scientific discovery is central to the theme of the book.

Emphasis is on the importance of diet, and lifestyle. Recommendation of a near zero carbohydrate intake is suggested for cancer patients. This, along with glutamine substituting drugs, or well known anti parasitic drugs, are crucial for a successful result in cancer remission.

Charles R Giardina

CONTENTS

PREFACE

This introductory section begins with a survey of the most important contents within the text. It emphasizes the last chapter of this document: A hard cancerous cell forgets how to die. Instead, the cell often multiplies thereby forming tumors. Worse yet, the cancerous cell can enter the blood stream and spread to other areas. Again, forming more tumors. This occurs when there is mitochondria dysfunction. Concurrently, the usual production process for energy creation changes. It transforms into a form of fermentation. That is, in cancerous cells energy production does not need Oxygen to power the cells, or tissues within the body. Therefore, the difference between normal cells and cancerous cells is how energy is produced.

Energy production for a cell is its most important function. This process is the conversion of potential energy, (the fuel) into kinetic energy. Fuel for a car is gasoline. The fuel for the mitochondria under cancerous conditions can only be glucose and glutamine. This was established by Warburg, in the 1920s, for glucose, that is for sugar, (Warburg, 1956). Also by Dr Seyfried, for the amino acid, glutamine, (Duraj, et al, 2024), (Lee, et al, 2024). Even recently it was thought that micro nutrients help cancerous growth. (Fagbohun, et al, 2023). But still glucose and glutamine are necessary and sufficient for continuation of the disease. (Seyfried, et al, 2025).

Several other substances are described in the last chapter, Chapter 4, all beneficial to cancer remission. Notably, Fenbendazole, a de-wormer, and Ivermectin, a parasitic. Both substances fight parasites. Parasites employ fermentation to create energy. There is a positive correlation between the use of both Fenbendazole and Ivermectin in conjunction with cancer fighting drugs. Cancer cells can only use fermentation to create energy. This is the deep correlation. Energy production, in the latter case, is through mitochondria substrate level phosphorylation in the glutaminolysis pathway.

Dr. Seyfried contends that Cancer is not a genetic disorder. Additionally, he contends semantic mutation theory is wrong. Mutations within the DNA are indicated with probabilities between [0,

1), but never equal to one. Abnormal diet and life style can lead to cancer. Toxic drugs in low dose may be okay for a person in a state of ketosis.

Beginning chapters of this document provide a background in mitochondria fundamentals. Additionally, they introduce basic principles of physics needed to understand chemical-biological changes within the body. The contents of these earlier chapters are briefly described next.

The first chapter provides an in-depth description of the mitochondria and its functions under normal conditions. Emphasis is on the energy creation methodology, provided in an in-depth manner. This enables a better understanding of energy production when cancer is present. Additional physics or chemical aspects are addressed in Appendix 1. Specifically, this involves the oxidation and reduction process. Also in the first chapter various aspects of the mitochondria dynamics are specified. In particular, a high, global view of the fission and fusion processes are explained and illustrated. Later chapters illustrate the operation of the fission or fusion process in providing treatments which produce cancer remission.

The second chapter describes the physics that are basic to all of the biological-chemical reactions within the body. Examples are provided, mainly with bodily elements, such as carbon, nitrogen, oxygen, etc. Additional elements, for instance, those useful for quantum dot production, are also specified. A description of quantum mechanical aspects ends this chapter. Quantum mechanics is the foundation for quantum tunneling in the mitochondria respiration system. Additionally, it is needed to fully understand properties of quantum dots.

The third chapter describes the process of ion creation, as well as the properties of nano particles. In particular, micro dots are illustrated, along with their use in medical applications. Appendix 2, gives the background of why quantum dots have a variety of colors. These colors range from red to blue. Instances of tunneling within the mitochondria are also provided in this chapter. Appendix 3, describes mathematical details for understanding the tunneling of particles.

1. THE MITOCHONDRIA

1.1 The Structure of Human Cells

There are a trillion cells within the body. These are the basic units of life and they are the smallest structural and functional living organisms. A cell is microscopic and is protected by a flexible surrounding membrane. Substances can selectively be transmitted into or out of the cell through the membrane. Most cells are eukaryotic cells. This means there is a nucleus interior to the cell, and rarely are there more than one. Within the nucleus there exists DNA. DNA is an abbreviation for the chemical Deoxyribo Nucleic Acid. The structure and purpose of this substance is described in Section 1.4.

All the material within a eukaryotic cell, with the exception of the nucleus is called the cytoplasm, or cytosol. It is a fluid, or jelly type material, within the material called a eukaryotic cell except for the organelles. These are small organs. There exists a nucleus membrane surrounding the nucleus. It is used for shielding it from the cytoplasm. Also, there exist protein complexes within the cytosol. However, the principle components within the liquid like cytoplasm are the organelles. The major type of organelles are the mitochondria. These are double walled structures. The interior of mitochondria is called the matrix.

Other small organs within the cytoplasm are cytoskeletons, which provide structure and firmness to the cell. Specifically, the cytoskeleton can hold the mitochondria within a certain region of the cell where they are most useful. The process is termed anchoring. Additionally, there are lysosome organelles within the cell, they act as recycling centers and play a role in cell death.

1.2 Mitochondria Structure and Basic Functions

About 99% of proteins within the mitochondria are transmitted from ribosomes located in the cytosol. They are mainly RNA, RiboNucleic Acid and are brought into the matrix using binding material. These ribosomes are often called cytosolic ribosomes. RNA are used in transcribing DNA into protein. Section 1.4, details the role of RNA in the transcription of DNA in creating proteins. The outer membrane of the mitochondria is porous, called porins, but the inner membrane is not porous. The one percent of proteins is manufactured in the matrix. The mtDNA encodes 13 proteins. The latter DNA refers to the mitochondria DNA.

Two types of metabolism are briefly mentioned. Catabolic energetic Adenosine TriphosPhate, ATP, which means breaking down complex molecules within a cell into less complex molecules, making energy. The energy component is ATP. Also anabolic biosynthetic, which means the build up complex molecules within a cell from less of complex molecules. The latter usually resorts to ATP energy for this transformation. ATP is formed with the help of the the Electron Transport Chain, ETC within the mitochondria. Figure 1.1 illustrates, but not to scale, the ETC within the mitochondria. Mitochondria not only produces energy in the form of ATP, but also it sends out the amino acid, serine. This substance transmits signals to create building blocks of protein.

Within the ETC there are about a hundred proteins. Approximately, 85% are controlled by the nucleus and the rest are controlled by the mitochondria. Mitochondria communicate by providing metabolites, which are molecules produced by metabolism. Communication occurs as well from its redox state. Here, there are large transfers of electrons that are described in more detail in Appendix 1. Mitochondria also have the ability to contact other organelles within the cell.

The Cristae refers to the folds within the inner membrane of the mitochondria. The wave like folding of the walls in the mitochondria increase its surface area. This is used for energy production. When cancer exists, the walls of the Cristae disappear. Cristae are illustrated in Figure 1.1.

Ribosomes located in the interior of the mitochondria inner boundary are proteins that are used in the process referred to as OXPHOS, or OXidative PHOSphorylation process. It translates information from the RNA to create amino acids, thereby forming proteins. These are the 13 proteins employed in the mtDNA, and ultimately used in the respiration process. Phosphorylation is the process of adding a phosphate molecule, PO_3, to another molecule. It can be thought to be an energy boosting enzyme. The molecule PO_3 consists of one atom of Phosphorus, P, and three atoms of Oxygen, O. The latter molecule is denoted by O_3, and sometimes by 3O. Section 2.5 provides basic facts and notations concerning molecules.

BAT is the Brown Adipose Tissue, which is in the mitochondria, and it also is illustrated in Figure 1.1. Its purpose is to regulate the heat within the cell by utilizing fatty acids and glucose for this production. In particular, in cold weather these BATs help keep the body warm. More information can be found in (Cedikova, et al, 2016). Interestingly enough there also exists in the mitochondria White Adipose Tissue, WAT, as well as beige Adipose Tissue, bAT. These are tissues which store and expend excess energy in the form of triglycerides droplets. Droplets regulate food intake and control lipid metabolism. See Section 1.5, for descriptions of different types of metabolic pathways. Enzymes enable the production of fatty acids as well as glycerols. The latter liquid substance is also known as glycerin and is a critical part of lipid acid.

WATs usually store fats, and BATs expend fats. Obesity occurs when more energy is stored than is utilized. Adipocyte, that is fat cells, can play a role in obesity. These occur by defects within the mitochondria in regulating the conversion of WATs to BATs.

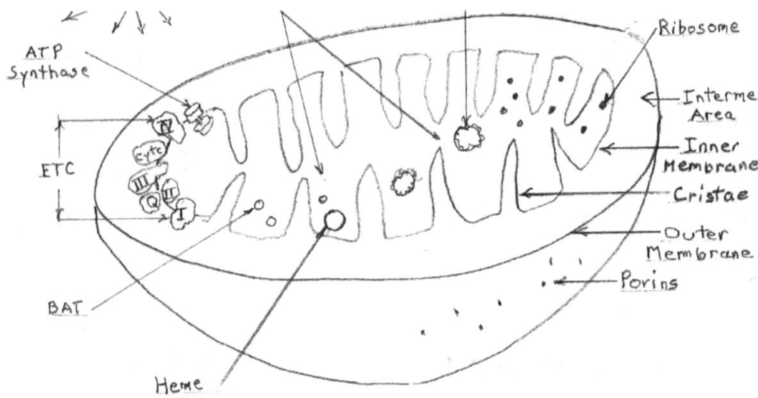

FIGURE 1.1) Mitochondria Structure

1 .3 Mitochondria Functionality And Pathology

Mitochondria perform four dynamic processes mobility, anchoring, fission and fusion. Contacts within a cell are temporal, and occur by tether proteins. This process could modify the resulting location of the mitochondria. The resulting position might be a distinct cell, for instance where more energy is needed. (Kraft, and Lockner, 2018).

Not only are the shape and position of a mitochondria important to cellular function, but so also is the actual anchoring. Anchoring determines the positioning and provides spatial, temporal, as well as contextual, control for the organelle. Mitochondria are strategically anchored within the cytoplasm to aid high energy demand locations. Anchoring is ensured using cytoskeletons. These organelles also locate mitochondria in order to optimize cell signaling. Moreover, they enhance the potential for producing fission and fusion. (Kraft, and Lackner, 2018).

The fission and fusion processes are illustrated in Figure 1.2. This diagram provides a high view of both the fission and fusion processes using a many sorted algebra type graph. Both processes involve only one sort, namely Mitochondria. This name is inscribed within the node of the graph.

For a succinct description of polyadic diagrams see, (Giardina, 2025). For the fission process, the polyadic arrow has a single tail, with two arrow head pointers. The polyadic arrow is labeled Drp1. It is illustrated in Figure 1.2. The mathematical meaning in this case is that Drp1 takes a single mitochondrion and makes two mitochondria. Actually, Drp1 is Dynamin-related protein 1; it is a helical ring located on the outer mitochondria membrane. It strangles, and severs the mitochondrion, producing two smaller ones.

The fusion process is the opposite of fission. The polyadic graph arrow has two tails, but has a single arrow head. It is labeled Opa1, meaning that this binary operator takes two mitochondria, and maps it into only one. It is illustrated in Figure 1.2B. Actually Opa1 is the protein, Optic atrophy 1. The actual biological process is more complicated, however the end result is the same. It involves first a fusion of the outer membranes, and subsequent fusion of the inner mitochondria membranes. See (Wang, et al, 2021), for more details

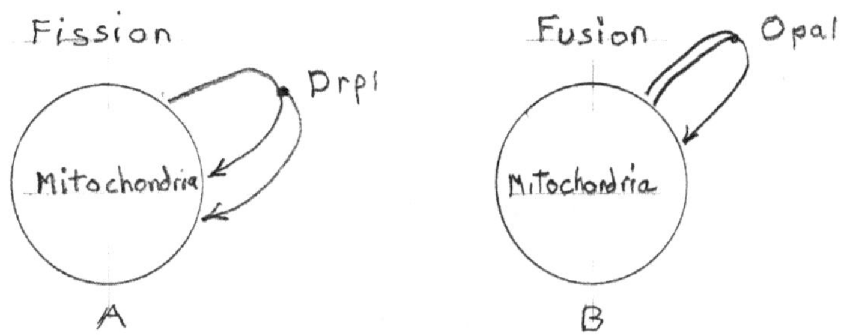

Figure 1.2) Polyadic Graphs for Fission and Fusion

Besides the creation of ATP, the mitochondria perform several other critical functions. These include:

- They help regulate Calcium levels within the body, this is important for muscle contraction and cell signaling.

- Mitochondria generate heat for the cells and the body.

- They perform fusion and fission processes . This is important in repairing mitochondrial dysfunction, and ensure cell cycling, as well as moderating cell death.

· The organelles send signaling molecules for balancing and moderating ROC, Reactive Oxygen Species, as well as calcium ions. The latter are calcium atoms containing a lesser, or greater number of electrons.

· They can metabolize fatty acids, as well organic compounds and amino acids.

· Mitochondria send signaling molecules for immunization, inflammation, as well as death indicators.

· They are involved in cell differentiation.

· The mitochondria can adapt to different environments, changes in nutrients as well as oxygen availability.

· They signal to other mitochondria, maintaining overall cellular wellness.

· Mitochondria have their own DNA.

· There is mitochondria communication inter as well as intra cell signaling.

- Mitochondria decide what part of a cell needs energy, and decides how much.

Section 1.4, provides an in-depth description of mtDNA, which are the specific mitochondria DNA. The DNA within the nucleus is also described in the referenced section, along with their large differences with mtDNA.

As previously mentioned, the mitochondria is not only the body's primary source for converting potential energy into kinetic energy, they also have numerous additional functions. They are essential for fatty acid oxidation. The mitochondria produces 95% of melatonin, and only 5%, or less is produced by the pineal gland in the brain. (Russel, et al, 2020) Most metabolically active organs and organelles contain the largest quantity of mitochondria. These organs include the heart, the brain, liver and kidneys. Oxidative respiration within the mitochondria has the largest influence on Reactive Oxygen Species, ROS. The mitochondria also control transcription of the DNA within the nucleus. They provide cell signaling as well as cell death, and play a primary role in aging. Aging is often associated with the accumulation of ROS, which is a byproduct of respiration.

Damage to the mitochondria can occur in numerous ways. There can be loss of mitochondria membrane integrity, or increased lipid peroxidation. The latter might be due to excessive omega six fatty acids. Fatty acids are associated with inflammation. Additionally, inflammation can cause mitochondria to die. Omega three help mitochondria to mitigate the negative effects of omega six. Further, there must be a balance between free radicals and antioxidants. Excessive ROS, that is insufficient antioxidants, is not beneficial. It is associated with an insufficient intake of trace minerals or green vegetables. When a deficiency exists there is damage to the tissue.

Surely, environmental aspects can greatly damage the mitochondria, such as toxins, pesticides, mycotoxins and Ionizing Radiation, IR. Microbiome imbalances are also cause for disfunction. For instance, fructose metabolism, produces MethyGlyOxal, MGO, which damages the mitochondria. MGO is known to contribute to numerous diseases, including cancer.

Mitochondria are major players in the overall health of a person. Among all eukaryotic cells about 90% of ROS is produced in the mitochondria ATP cycle. ROS helps regulate cellular redox stress, and breaks down metabolites of high energy as well as regulating cell death. It is essential for cell immunity. However, excessive ROS is associated with the proliferation and survival of many cancers. (Sabbarwal, and Schumacher, 2014).

Fission and fusion processes are constantly occurring depending upon the cells requirements. But these processes are disrupted by immune related inflammatory diseases. When this occurs, stress increases the fission process and decreases mitochondria fusion. (Fang, et al, 2024). Section 4.3 illustrates mitochondria undergoing the fission and fusion process. The carrier set in this situation is pancreatic cancer mitochondria. Drugs are applied to produce fusion and thereby inhibit the cancerous spread.

On the other hand, when T cells are concerned, the roles of fission and fusion might be reversed. T cells protect the body from pathologies with the help of B cells which make antibodies. T cells with the immunity property are enhanced by the genetic fusion process. The process improves their cancer fighting abilities. This is particularly important in opposing solid tumors. (Lanna, and Dustin, 2016). However, the next document, (Cleveland Clinic, 2025), details the benefits of the fission protocol.

In short, the fission process refers to the process of splitting an entity into two entities, and fusion refers to the combining of two entities into a single one. The mitochondria is the energy source for cells within the body. Finally, it should be mentioned that quantum tunneling exists in both the fission and fusion processes. For a description of quantum tunneling see, (Giardina, 2024). In nuclear fission, some radioactive particles of the alpha type tunnel through potential energy barriers involving the nucleus of an isotope. All types of fusion involving the mitochondria, usually involve quantum tunneling. Fusion may also alter the DNA indirectly by causing free radicals to form. Specifically, the body is made up of mostly water, and contact with these particles or waves could modify the water atoms. In this case H_2O molecules are transformed into the following molecules:

Hydrogen, H; Also hydroxyls, OH; As well as hydrogen superoxide, HO_2; Additionally, H_2, dihydrogen: Or even hydrogen peroxide, H_2O_2. (NRC.gov, 2014). The absolute amount of radiation released in nuclear sources is inversely proportional to the half life of the radiating source.

Mitochondrial dysfunction is analyzed in (Morris, and Berk, 2015), The many roads to mitochondrial dysfunction in neuraimmune and neuropsychiatric disorders, is addressed in (BMC Med, 2015). There is a high correlation between loss of membrane integrity and increased lipid per oxidation. Lipid peroxidation indicates excessive omega six fatty acids and not enough omega three. See, (Schuster, et al, 2018) for more details. Excessive ROS correlates with a lack of antioxidants. In the mitochondria, Manganese SuperOxide Dismutase, MnSOD, protects cells from oxidative stress. For instance, in the gut, microbial infections are prevented by MnSOD. In particular MnSOD resists the presence of ROS.

Fructose produces methylglyoxal, which destroys mitochondrial capacity. It is a damaging agent for metabolism. Also, it is an aging agent as well as a diabetes inducing agent. Additionally, methylglyoxal harms gene transcription. See (Nigro, C et al, 2019), and (Gugliucci, A, et al, 2017) Finally, methylglyoxal is shown to cause a fatty liver.

Environmental factors involving pesticides, mycotoxins as mold, as well as ionizing radiation, are damaging agents for the mitochondria. For an in-depth description of the latter damaging agent see (Giardina, 2025).

Cellular metabolism and health integrity of cells are regulated by the mitochondria. There exist on average about 2000 mitochondria within a cell ,occupying from one-twentieth to one-quarter of the volume. Each mitochondrion converts potential energy into kinetic energy. The potential energy involves glucose, oxygen, water as well as amino acids, and fatty acids. The kinetic energy is used to power the cells along with enabling inter and intra cell signaling of other mitochondria, and as a heat source. Where more energy is needed, as in muscle cells, hundreds of thousand sof mitochondria can exists within each cell. Using electronic transport signaling, they produce

ATP, referring to the site of oxidative phosphorylation. ATP is the energy generated.

Cells increase the number of mitochondria during cell growth as well as giving rise to fission, the property of splitting apart. This was previously mentioned earlier in this section along with fusion. Recall that the latter refers to two distinct mitochondria joining together to form an elongated interconnected structure, and sharing their information. Fission and fusion can be considered as two aspects of mitochondria quality control. In particular, fission can be thought of as a repair process. Fission byproducts are the creation of normal mitochondria. (Su, et al, 2023).

Some reports say that the lens within the eyes, as well as red blood cells have no mitochondria. (Lenzen, 2014), (Helmenstine, 2024). On the other hand, some scientists found mitochondria within human blood. (Lazaro, 2025).

1.4 DNA In the Nucleus and in the Mitochondria

DNA is a chemical polymer. That is, it is a large molecule comprised of many smaller molecules.

DNA is organized in a double helix type ladder structure, and its normal state consists of a compactly constructed formation. DNA are compressed to fit within the nucleus of a cell. If untangled, a single DNA strand is about six feet in length, and consists of 46 sections or chromosomes. However, only 23 different types of DNA exist and each appears as a compressed spring. The two chromosomes which are the same are called chromosome pairs. Each pair is created by both the mother and the father. The last pair are called the sex chromosomes. If the last chromosome pair is XY, then it is indicative of a male. When this pair is XX, this denotes a female. Genes are short segments of chromosomes that provide code for a specific gene.

Genome is the entire set of genetic material. Amino acids are chemical molecules within the body that combine to form proteins. In short, they break down food and create proteins. There are about twenty types of amino acids having distinct shapes. Amino acids consist of atoms: Oxygen, O; Carbon, C; Hydrogen, H; Nitrogen, N. Sometimes; Sulfur, S; Phosphorous, P. Additionally, ions from these atoms often also appear. Amino acids exist within the cell in the cytoplasm. DNA provides a script for how the amino acids should combine to provide specific proteins. There are millions of different proteins. Each consists of a polypeptite chain of amino acids. A strand of DNA is made up of millions of nucleotides. These are building blocks for both DNA and RNA, and are detailed below.

Transcription occurs by making partial copies of DNA, called RNA. RNA look like DNA but are shorter length strings, and they consist of one side of the ladder structure. The nucleotides are in the case of RNA, labeled A, G, C, and U. In order, these labels are abbreviations for the following acid bases, adenine, guanine, cytosine and uracil, respectively. These occur mainly in the nucleus. They travel to the cytoplasm, and because they are narrow, they can pass through pours in the nucleus and through the boundary of the cytoplasm. Subsequently, they appear in the ribosome. It is here that protein is created three letters at a time. This construct is referred to as a codon.

Cells within the body consists of three parts, the cell membrane which forms the exterior boundary, the inner annuli part called the cytoplasm, and the innermost nucleus. As previously mentioned, the cytoplasm refers to the fluid which fills the cell, but it also includes proteins and amino acids as well as organelles. The nucleus is the cell's control center. Most of the time, it is here that the DNA exists. Four acid bases exist within the DNA. They are abbreviated C, G, A, and T. The first three were specified previously, and the fourth basis is thymine. These are chemically composed of sugar and phosphate molecules. Therefore, they consist of H, O, C and N. They appear as a sequence within a double helix spiral comprising the DNA. The pairings are A and T, also G and C. See Figure 1.3A.

Phosphate forms the backbone of DNA. Chromosomes carry the DNA within the nucleus of the cell when the nucleus exists. A small amount of DNA appears in the mitochondria. This DNA is abbreviated as mtDNA. As noted, mitochondria convert potential energy into kinetic energy. This happens within all cells except possibly not in blood cells. As mentioned above, mtDNA compresses in order to fit within a cell's nucleus. Specifically, this string is tightly wrapped around numerous histones. Histones are described in more depth next.

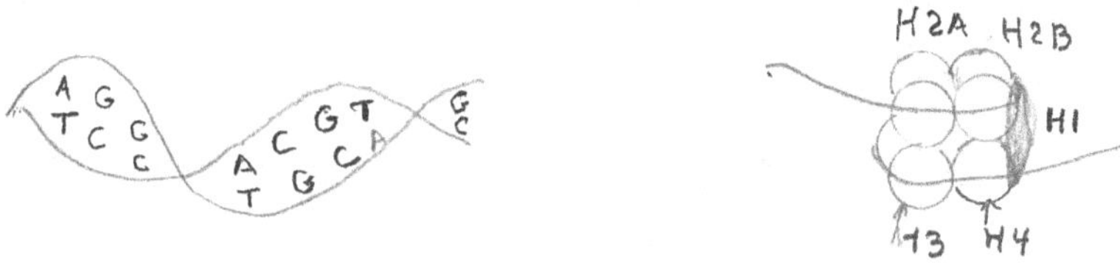

A B

FIGURE 1.3) DNA and Histone Modification

All cells within a human body contain the same DNA sequence, however there are distinct epigenetic modifications within a cell. Epigenetic processes are employed in interpreting DNA. Epigenetic means on top of genetics. The term refers to external interpretation of the DNA. It turns genes on and off and describes changes in gene expression which are not encoded within the actual DNA sequence. These modifications do not change the DNA sequence but involve various types of epigenetic regulators to describe gene transcription. These are non-coded RNA, also more specifically methylation modification, and histone modification.

Methylation modification and histone modification enable the creation of distinct cell types, such as skin, kidney, muscle and so on. They also prohibit certain modifications to occur, and might reverse previously made modifications. Epigenetic modifications occur as a result of aging, drugs, diet, and environment; in particular in reaction to toxins such as ionizing radiation.

RNA polymerase, that is RiboNucleic Acid Polymerase, RNAP, is an enzyme which, with the help of other proteins, binds itself to a specific part of the DNA. It provides the transcription process. This is itself a catalyst, and needs no starting or stopping conditions. (B D Editors, 2019). In short, the transcription process maps DNA into RNA and this is translated into proteins. The mappings are:

DNA———>RNA———->Protein.

DNA methylation is the process in which DNA is not in the active state; transcription cannot be performed.

Methylation modification is the process by which methyl molecules attache themselves to DNA.

This is the normal state, occurring 75% of the time. A methyl molecule consists of a carbon atom which bonds with three hydrogen atoms. When present, this prevents certain gene expression from turning on or turning off. When the methyl molecule is attached, it usually attaches to C or G, also called a CpG island. This occurs because C and G have more bonds, namely three, instead of two for A or T. High DNA methylation ensures inactivate DNA transcription. It is a defense mechanism. Un-methylation DNA can make cancer or bacteria more likely. In short, high methylation prevents RNA from forming, thus

DNA—-x—>RNA—x—>protein.

Histones have interior units as well as an exterior structure, with the latter histone designated H1. H1 is the largest unit and the most important protein. It holds the interior units together. It binds the Histones and enables DNA, with condensed wrapping needed to be contained within the nucleus. The interior histone units have two of each H2A, H2B, H3, and H4 protein. See Figure 1.3B. Histones are positively charged and this enhances the binding with the negatively charged DNA. Modifications do occur, which involves epigenetic factors which relax the tightly wound DNA. This can be thought of as the open state and it is called histone acetylation. It enables proteins to be read from the genes. DNA that are tightly wrapped around histones cannot be read by the cell. This can be thought of as the more usual common closed state. De-acetylation makes transcription much less possible because the DNA is wrapped tightly. When the chromosome is relaxed, there is a higher chance of cancer occurring. Over acting de-acetylation leads to gene silencing, it cannot transcribe at all. In short, de-acetylation prevents DNA from being transformed into RNA, so,

DNA —-x—>RNA—-x—->protein.

Genes are sequences of DNA. Specifically, and as previously mentioned, a codon is a triple of base elements. Gene mutation can occur when one nucleotide is changed, inserted or deleted, producing an erroneous protein. (Tatomir, 2024). Living organisms have genes which determine the composition of amino acids and proteins within the body.

A simple type of mutation is described next. It involves low frequency UV light of wave length 120 nano meters, 120nm to 400 nano meters, 400nm. Nucleotides, Thymine and Cytosine, that is T and C cross linking, forms a kink in the DNA, and the RNA cannot be formed. A consequence is that transcription becomes impossible. In this case, protein cannot stop dividing the cell due to mutation.

Mitochondria contain their own DNA. This DNA is denoted as mtDNA. Its purpose is similar to the DNA within the nucleus of a cell. The mtDNA is double stranded and is formed as a circular molecule with base pairs. There are an average of two thousand mitochondria within a cell, each having one to ten strands of mtDNA. However, there are two more striking differences from DNA. First, only the mother's DNA is utilized in mtDNA structure. More importantly, is that the histone protection described previously for the nucleus DNA is totally absent in the mtDNA. A consequence is that in the natural state, the closed state of protected DNA is not present in mtDNA. The latter DNA is not histone tightly compressed, it is wide open inviting Ionizing Radiation, IR, to hit it. This open state makes the mtDNA is more vulnerable to damaging agents. Mitochondrial dysfunction can arise from IR and the result can be cancer. The mtDNA is illustrated in Figure 1.1.

The effect of IR can be better understood in relation to the process by which ATP is transmitted. Indeed, signals are sent using the ETC within the mitochondria. This chain is comprised of protein clusters. The protein clusters transfer electrons through membranes within the mitochondria. The overall goal is the creation of kinetic energy in the form of ATP. It occurs by the formation of a proton gradient. The process is called OXPHOS, and is described in more detail in Section 1.6, and Appendix 1. The number of ETC within the mitochondria depends heavily on the cell's function. The heart mitochondria have 30,000 sets of ETC, whereas the liver has one third that amount. (Sapkota, 2024).

During OXPHOS, between one percent to five percent of electrons leak out the mitochondria's boundaries. These are the inner and outer membranes. The outer membrane can allow ions to penetrate, whereas the inner membrane is almost impermeable to ion crossings. The space in-between is called the inter membrane area and is part of the mitochondria as is the matrix. The latter is the area within the inner membrane. The actual process involved in ETC is described in Section 1.6.

When an atom gains one or more electrons it is called an anion. On the other hand, if it loses an electron and becomes positively charged it is called a cation. These are the two distinct types of charged ions. In metabolic type processes there are present free radicals, which are positively charged ions, that is, they are cations. Anti-oxidants cling to positive radicals, resulting in non charged molecules. Anti-oxidants are anions. During cellular respiration small amounts of free radicals escape the mitochondria. They can attack protein lipids in blood cells, as well as in DNA. This results in cell damage and can cause cancer. A common occurrence is when there are too many free radicals. The overall process is called oxidative stress.

Mitochondria dysfunction effects DNA transcription, translation, regulation of expression and protein activation. Additionally, the mtDNA has less ability for self repair than nuclear DNA. Mitochondria have 37 genes encoding for 13 proteins. These all are involved in OXPHOS. Furthermore, mitochondria have little or no repair type genes nor do they have proliferative type genes. (Leija, et al, 2017).

1.5 Metabolic Pathways

Metabolic pathways refers to chemical and physics type reactions within a human cell. In this document, physics is emphasized because all reactions involve electrons, protons, and generalizations of atoms in all cases. Several metabolic pathways are described herein. They function within an eukaryotic cell. An excellent reference is (Creative Proteomics, 2025). This article is especially good at describing the Pentose Phosphate Pathway, PPP, process summarized below along with its relationship with glycolysis.

· Glycolysis - the brain is 2% of body's weight , but consumes 20% of the body's oxygen consumption and 60% of glucose intake. The brain also uses amino acids, fatty acids or lactate for providing energy. However, it lacks fuel storing ability. The Warburg effect, initiated in the 1920s, specified that cancer is caused by mitochondria dysfunction. It involves the increased glucose consumption by the cancerous tumor. Additionally, there is a conversion of glucose to lactate outside the mitochondria as opposed to byproducts of the OXPHOS process. However, the human brain uses about ten percent of glucose produced by non oxidative metabolism that is aerobic glycolysis.

· Lipid Metabolism, occurs when a cell's glucose supplies are low. Lipids are usually not so soluble in water. They are an alternate energy source. In general, lipid metabolism breaks down fats as its source of energy. This can only occur in a non-cancerous cell. Cells store fats as triglycerides and lipid metabolism converts triglycerides into glycerol and fatty acids. After this, glycerol enters the glycolysis pathway then it goes into the Krebs cycle. A description of the Krebs cycle, and related remarks, are found in Section 1.6. Fatty acids are converted into acetyl Coenzyme A, also called acetyl CoA, or just CoA. This is produced by beta oxidation. CoA is a molecule which is instrumental in beginning ATP energy production by allowing entry into the matrix. As in the glycolysis metabolism, CoA also proceeds into the Krebs cycle. Subsequently, outputs from the Krebs cycle help perform OXPHOS. Ketones are a byproduct of lipid metabolism.

· Pentose Phosphate Pathway, PPP-this pathway produces the molecule NADPH, Nicotinamide Adenine Dinucleotide Phosphate in an oxidative stage. PPP also creates ribose five phosphate. The overall purpose of PPP is to provide nucleotide synthesis. As previously mentioned, these are building blocks for both DNA and RNA. PPP has other important purposes such as decreasing oxidative stress, and it is useful for redox reactions. See Appendix 1, describing redox reaction in greater detail. The PPP process does not directly produce ATP.

1.6 Aerobatic Respiration in Healthy Cells

Aerobic cellular respiration is the normal process whereby cells of the body break down glucose to form energy ATP. This process involves molecules of oxygen. Oxygen must be present even at the end of the ATP generation, otherwise the process would be stopped. The waste products are both carbon dioxide and water. This is in contrast to anaerobic cellular respiration, wherein oxygen is not employed in the energy creation. Other electron acceptors like sulfate are employed. Moreover, in anaerobic cellular respiration, the yield of ATP is much less than in aerobic cellular respiration. Furthermore, waste products are lactic acid as well as ethanol, in this case. The anaerobic type of respiration is described in Section 4.1, involving cancer.

For live humans, aerobic cellular respiration is a closed loop system. The person has enough energy to take in food, including carbohydrate nutrients or proteins, which are ultimately converted into glucose. Subsequently, excretions, including carbon dioxide and water, are formed. There are four steps in the process of breaking down and converting ATP into Adenosine DiPhosphate ADP, and then reversing the process. These conversions occur about 300 times each day. (Sapkota, 2024). Next, a short description is provided for each step in the aerobatic respiration process. Then this is followed by more in depth details.

· Glycolysis - In this the first step, glucose is broken down into two molecules of pyruvate. This occurs in the cytoplasm. Pyruvate acts like a fuel, inducing entry into the Krebs cycle within the mitochondria. During this process a small amount of ATP, along with molecules of Nicotinamide Adenine Dinucleotide, NADH are produced. This occurs from pyruvate oxidation. As mentioned before, the glycolysis process takes place in the cytoplasm, and does not need oxygen. It is the lack of oxygen which enables glycolysis, a fundamental agent for cancerous tumor growth.

· Krebs Cycle - This is the second stage for healthy cells. Pyruvate is converted into acetal CoA allowing its actual entry into the mitochondria and initiating the Krebs cycle. This process results in releasing energy and CO_2 as waste. It also produces more NADH as well as molecules of Flavin Adenine Dinucleotide, $FADH_2$. Numerous steps within the cycle convert the ion NAD^+ into NADH. The whole process occurs within the mitochondria matrix.

· ETC - Now for the third step in the aerobatic respiration process. Four stages of protein complexes store potential energy utilizing electrons lost from molecules NADH and $FADH_2$. This results in a proton gradient. It is a transformation utilizing great amounts of H^+ molecules. These are protons located in the matrix. They flow into the mitochondria inter membrane area. A proton gradient is formed. That is, the ETC process produces a much higher concentration of proton charges within the inter membrane area than in the matrix.

At the end of the process water, H_2O, and carbon dioxide CO_2, are created from the end stage, which is oxygen. If oxygen was not present then ETC could not function. The whole ETC process exists within the matrix and the inter membrane area. Its purpose is to create the proton gradient previously mentioned.

· Chemiosmosis - This is the final step, Here the ATP is actually generated much like in a windmill, in a hydro plant or in a nuclear reactor. They all employ a turbine to produce energy. Instead of wind or water to cause centripetal motion, here the proton flow is the source of motion. This is due to the proton gradient. A large difference with turbine generation of electricity is that in the chemiosmosis process, it is a digital process. More precisely, the implementation is a discrete step wise process. Protons go into the mitochondria matrix, exiting from the fluid filled inter membrane space one at a time. The movement is due to the large gradient between the density of protons in the inter mitochondria membrane and the matrix of the mitochondria.

The following is a more in-depth, step-by-step description of aerobatic respiration under non diseased conditions.

The First Stage <u>Glycolysis</u>

Glucose enters the body and goes through one of four GLUcose Transformers, GLUTs, to enter specific tissues. This occurs with the help of enzymes. Actually there are two transporters, the primary is GLUT, and the secondary is SGLT, standing for Sodium GLUcose Transport. GLUT is bidirectional, meaning it is a two way path; substances entering can be returned from inside a cell to the outside again. However, SGLT is unidirectional. The latter utilizes electrochemical gradients across plasma membranes as energy. Only GLUT will be described herein.

There are fourteen different GLUTs, however, only five are well characterized. Moreover, they do not rely on ATP for their function. They distribute glucose everywhere in various tissues throughout the body. They direct the glucose to the pancreas, small intestines, neurons in the brain, skeletal muscles, white blood cells, the spleen, the liver, and so on.

Since GLUT is bidirectional, a prevention mechanism is introduced to prevent glucose from returning to the source. This is performed by two enzymes which create a chemical reaction within the tissue. Actually, the mechanism occurs by attaching a phosphate group to the sixth carbon molecule within the glucose molecule. The phosphate group is an ionic molecule, the anion, PO_4^{3-}. The molecule ADP is a precursor to ATP. When ATP loses the phosphate group, PO_4^{3-}, it returns to ADP. PO_4^{3-} is a molecule containing one Phosphorous, P atom. It also possesses a single Oxygen atom along with three Oxygen ions.

Actually, ten steps occur in the Glycolysis process, that is, in the conversion of glucose into two molecules of pyruvate. The first five phases consume energy by using two molecules of ATP, but the last five phases gain four molecules of ATP as well as two molecules of NADH. The latter substance is needed in the ETC stage. So within the Cytosol, by using glycolysis a net gain of two ATP energy units are manufactured.

It should be mentioned that substances other than glucose can be broken down, allowing entry in to the next stage, the Krebs cycle. These substances are fatty acids and ketone bodies. This is achieved using β-Oxidation. Section 4.1, specifies that this method only works for healthy cells. Cancerous cells cannot utilize these substances as potential energy. Similarly, glutaminolysis can break down various amino, or glucagenic, or ketogenic acids. The description of the Krebs cycle below initially emphasizes the glycolysis process.

Krebs Cycle

The Krebs, or TriCarboxylic Acid, TCA, cycle begins in the mitochondria matrix. This occurs from the previous stage by introducing two molecules of pyruvate into the cytosol. (Biology LibreTexts, 2014). Recall, that pyruvate is created from glucose in the first part of the respiration process, the glycolysis stage. Additionally, two molecules of ATP and two molecules of NADH are also created. Before the actual cycle begins, Pyruvate can be metabolized and converted to Acetyl CoA. However, it can also be converted into Alanine, or Lactic acid. It also can produce Oxaloacetate. The substances Alanine, or Lactic acid, can be reconverted into two molecules of Pyruvate.

In order to continue with the usual respiration process, assume that pyruvate produces Acetyl CoA. Then with the help of a transport protein, Acetyl CoA enters both the outer and inner walls of the mitochondria matrix. Concurrently it also creates 2 NADH molecules.

Starting the cycle, is Acetyl CoA. With this initial condition, Acetyl CoA—->Citrate, and the cycle begins: Citrate—->Isocitrate—*—>Alpha-Ketoglutarate—*—>Succinyl-CoA—->Succinate —#—>Fumarate——>Malate—*—>Oxaloacetate —->Citrate, and the cycle ends, and begins again. The stars (*) indicate locations where three high energy NADH molecules are generated. The symbol (#) denotes the location where one molecule of high energy FADH2 molecule is created. These molecules are needed in the ETC where they will provide electrons for proton pumping. ADP enhances the Krebs cycle, but ATP inhibits the cycle. Some ROS is also created in this stage. However, a net result of two ATP units are gained from this step.

ETC Stage

The ETC stage is mainly designed to produce a very large proton charge within the inter membrane space of the mitochondria. It occurs by using three protein complexes that are bound to the inner mitochondria membrane. The large proton charge is acquired from the proton source in the mitochondria matrix. The actual transfer of protons from the matrix utilizes electrons provided by the high energy NADH, and FADH2 molecules, originally acquired in the Krebs cycle. These electrons pass through a sequence of redox reactions within protein complexes. See Appendix 1. By doing so, energy is released, thereby forming a proton gradient and thus enabling the transfer of protons.

The architecture involving the ETC is comprised of four large protein complexes. These are specified by Roman numerals: I, NADH-CoQ Reductase; II, Succinate Dehydrogenase; III, Cytochrome bc1 Complex; IV, Cytochrome Oxidase. These proteins are used in pumping the protons from inside the mitochondria, that is from the matrix. They go to the destination, the area between the inner membrane and outer membrane. This space is called the inter membrane area. Ultimately, by producing a higher concentration of positive charges within the inter membrane area than in the matrix, a gradient is formed.

Specifically, only proteins I, III, and IV directly pump protons out of the matrix. Protons go thru the membrane from one side to the other. Protein II only aids in the pumping. In Figure 1.4, there exists a diagram of the ETC and also the ATP synthase. The complexes, and other structures are not drawn to scale. This diagram is supposed to be a magnification of the ETC portion of Figure 1.1. On the left side is the ETC and the ATP synthase. Four complexes are identified. These are in order, complex I, II, III, and IV, and constitute the ETC. Following these complexes is the ATP synthase block. All these structures make up the electron and proton reactions ultimately leading to the OXPHOS production of ATP. The final ATP production stage is also called chemiosmosis.

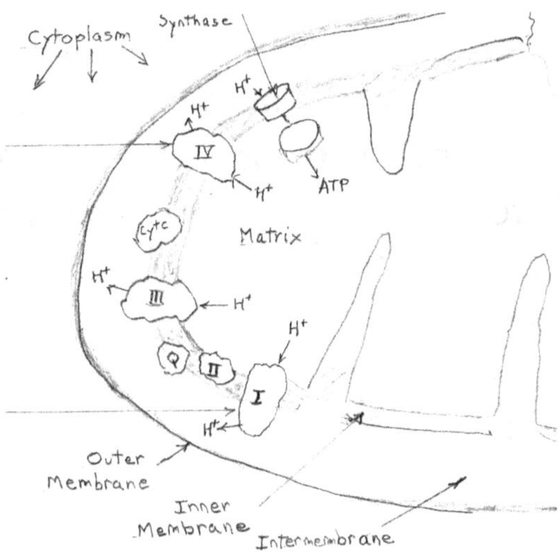

FIGURE 1.4) ETC and Chemiosmosis Process

In between complexes I, and III is complex II, as well as the Coenzyme Q, CoQ block. Between III and IV is the CytC block. The CoQ is a lipid electron transporter. It is an abbreviation for Coenzyme Q, and sends electrons to complex III. The CytC block is short for Cytochrome C, which is a water soluble protein located within the inter membrane area. It shuttles electrons from complex III to complex IV. Beginning in the mitochondrial matrix there exist protons labeled H^+. These protons will be transferred to the inter membrane space. As NADH approaches complex I, it becomes the cation molecule, NAD^+. Additionally, it releases electrons to complex I. This is the first enzyme within the ETC, it also contains bacteria. Because of the negative charge in complex I, this protein becomes super-charged and attracts protons from the matrix. Accordingly, protons are pumped from the matrix into the inter membrane space. Concurrently, complex I, sends electrons to the CoQ block.

Simultaneously, molecules of FADH2 enter the ETC. Similarly, this molecule becomes a cation molecule. Symbolically, FADH-->FAD^+, these lost electrons enter complex II. Electrons within complex II are then sent to CoQ, also known as the Q pool. After this, CoQ sends electrons to complex III. This process supercharges complex

III. It transmits additional protons from the matrix into the inter membrane space. Also, complex III sends electrons to CytC which subsequently sends electrons to complex IV.

Again, as in complexes I, and III, complex IV is supercharged and pumps protons from the matrix into the inter membrane space. Simultaneously, however, in this case complex IV passes its electrons to oxygen. This last step occurs only if oxygen is present, meaning that the human is still capable of inhaling oxygen. By accepting electrons, oxygen splits into two oxygen ions. Subsequently, these ions form two water molecules. This ends the ETC stage, the outputs are waste water, and CO_2. (Ahmad, 2023). The water waste is exhaled from a humans breath along with the carbon dioxide, mainly manufactured in the Krebs cycle.

Chemiosmosis Stage

The proton concentration gradient forces a single proton from the inner mitochondria membrane into the upper part of the ATP synthase. Concurrently, another proton leaves the synthase and arrives at the lower ATP synthase. This structure is part of the mitochondria matrix. The upper part of the synthase rotates to enable another proton to enter. After several protons have entered, this process ensures enough energy is created. The energy is utilized in the bottom part of the ATP synthase. Here, oxidative phosphorylate transforms ADP into ATP. The ATP stores energy for the human body.

The molecule, ADP is a precursor to ATP. When ATP loses the phosphate group, PO_4^{3-}, it returns to being ADP. Previously mentioned, the phosphate group consists of a single Phosphorous atom, P surrounded by a single Oxygen atom O, and three Oxygen anions. These three structures are Oxygen ions with an additional electron attached to each.

Production of a high density of positive charges in the inter membrane space compared to the lessor density of positive charge in the matrix, enables the ATP production. OXPHOS begins in the ETC. The ETC drives the ATP cycle by utilizing a proton gradient arising from energy of electrons stored within acceptors.

Finally, because of the magnitude of protons in the inter membrane space, and a lesser amount within the matrix, a proton gradient is formed. The gradient forces protons to travel into the matrix with the help of the conversion of ADP into ATP in the synthase. This is how the energy is formed. Simultaneously, the closed loop cycle continues by creating NADH and FADH2 and sending them back to the complexes. Between the ETC and the Chemiosmosis step a net total of 34 ATP units are created.

The last two steps in the aerobic cellular respiration process are called Oxidative Phosphorylation OXPHOS. A more in-depth description of OXPHOS is described in Appendix 1. It utilizes some concepts from Chapter 2. Additionally, glucose is hoarded by cancer cells since they only obtain 2ATP units from the Glycolysis process, instead of 34 ATP units during OXPHOS.

1.7 Toxins Inhibiting The Aerobic Respiration Processes

· Rotenone - This substance is often used as a pesticide, and it is poorly absorbed by the skin. However, oral intake can be fatal. It inhibits complex I during the ETC process by blocking the flow of electrons.

· Antimycin A - This is known as a piscicide, that is, it's a chemical substance which is a toxic poison for fish. It is harmful in complex III by preventing the electron transport to CoQ.

· Cyanide - Known as a highly toxic agent, CN^- is also often used in the manufacturing of plastics and rubber products. It acts similar to antimycin A, but instead inhibits complex IV.

· Carbon Monoxide CO - This gas disrupts the ETC process, mainly by preventing complex IV functionality.

· Oligomycin - Along with being a well known anti-bacterial agent, it is poisonous to humans. It harms ATP synthase, that is the final OXPHOS stage, chemiosmosis. Oligomycin acts like an uncoupling agent, it prohibits proton passage into the matrix.

2. QUANTUM BIOLOGY AND CHEMISTRY

2.1 Outline of The Chapter

What are referred to as bonds between molecules within the body, or even the conversion of matter into energy, are both quantum mechanical effects. The same is true for light absorption, along with the cellular respiration process. To better understand the human body and its composition, basic structures are reviewed. This begins in Section 2.2, where the Hydrogen atom, H is discussed, along with its atomic structure. In the next section energy and electron structures for the most prevalent elements within the body are described. These include: Carbon, C; Nitrogen, N; Oxygen, O; Phosphorous P; Sulfur, S.

Bonds between molecules often involve ions of atoms. This concept is described and illustrated in Section 2.4. Examples are provided for those life essential elements as well as other elements, such as Cadmium and Selenium. The latter elements are referenced in a later chapter involving the use of micro devices in organ dysfunction detection and their cure. The next section is concerned with molecular bonding along with ionic bonding. Various examples are provided for elements within the body as well as those elements which are toxic. Section 2.6, gives a brief description of excitons and the exciton Bohr Radius. The important concept of energy gap is described in this section.

The final section in this chapter is very different from the other sections. Whereas, the other sections are often referred to as quantum chemistry, this section is one hundred percent quantum mechanics. It is needed in order to provide the background for understanding quantum dots, illustrated on the cover of this text. These dots are useful in the detection process of tissue disfunction as well as aiding in remedies. Additionally, this section provides the basics for understanding the underlying quantum tunneling effect within the mitochondria.

2.2 Basic Structure of Atoms and Their Isotopes

All atoms are arranged containing a nucleus forming the center, and always have at least one proton. Protons are positively charged within the nucleus of the atom. The number of protons within an atom is called the atomic number n, of the element. These numbers are recorded and identify unique atoms. This is documented in an orderly fashion all within the Periodic Table of Elements, PTE. Every atom, except Hydrogen, H with an atomic number one, also has neutrons within the nucleus of the atom. Both protons and neutrons are about equal in mass. Here these masses are normalized, and called one atomic mass. Whereas, protons have a positive charge, neutrons are uncharged particles.

Additionally, there exist electrons of negative charge always moving in a circular motion about the nucleus within electron shells. Centripetal force necessary for revolution exists due to the electrostatic force involving the attraction between neutrons and electrons. With the orbiting of the electrons, the atom appears of large volume, but the entire mass essentially exists within the nucleus. It is said that the nucleus has 99.9% of the mass within an atom. Accordingly, herein the electrons are assumed to be of zero atomic mass. The atomic mass of an atom is the sum of the number of protons plus the number of neutrons. An atom that is said to be neutral has the number of protons which equals the number of electrons. Consequently, saying that an atom is neutral also means that the overall atom does not have a non zero charge.

An illustration of a neutral atom, a Hydrogen atom of mass one is illustrated in Figure 2.1 A). There exists a single electron continually orbiting in a three dimensional electron shell. A single proton exists within the nucleus.

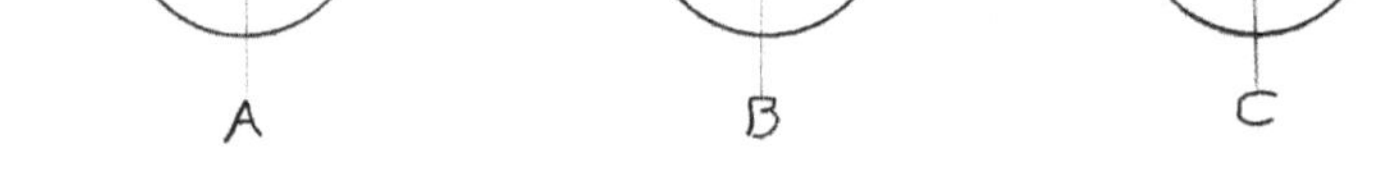

FIGURE 2.1) Hydrogen Atom and Isotopes

The number of neutrons within an atom is variable, and the number of neutrons only changes the atomic mass number. A specific atom with atomic number n, can have various, usually a large amount of neutrons. Sometimes less neutrons than protons. These resulting structures are called isotopes. In the actual PTE the atomic mass is listed for a specific atom, and it is the average of all its isotopes masses. The number of isotopes associated with an atom can be very large. However, many of these isotopes are unstable. Even though these isotopes are unstable, they share similar chemical properties, but they have radioactive decay. Radioactive decay is the process of influencing the isotopes to become more stable. In unstable isotopes the result is often the creation of a different atom. In any case, the half life of such a particle characterizes about the time it takes for an isotope to lose half of its radioactivity.

In Figure 2.1, three isotopes of Hydrogen, H are illustrated, there exist other isotopes of H. However, these three are found in the environment. In Figure 2.1A is the usual Hydrogen atom existing in the largest percentage of 99.8 %. It is sometimes called protium and symbolized by 1H, or by $^{1}_{1}H$. In the latter symbology the upper one indicates the atomic mass = 1, and the lower one indicates the atomic number = 1.

Figure 2.1B is another stable Hydrogen isotope called Deuterium. It has a neutron within the nucleus, as well as the one proton. It is denoted by, ${}_{1}^{2}H$, since its atomic mass is two. Finally, Figure 2.1C, illustrates the Hydrogen isotope Tritium, ${}_{1}^{3}H$. This means that besides one proton there exist two additional neutrons within the nucleus. The latter isotope is not stable and has a half life of 12.32 years. Several additional isotopes of Hydrogen exist, but they are created in the laboratory, and they are very unstable. (Jolly, 2025).

2.3 Structure of Atoms, Electron Configuration

The Bohr model of an atom describes how electrons are arranged in a circular fashion about the center nucleus. These are called energy configuration diagrams. Even though atoms are three dimensional, and several orbits are not exactly circular, concentric circles are used in two dimensional diagrams. A simple example is provided in Figure 2.1. An additional example is provided in Figure 2.2A, where a Helium atom is illustrated. In this diagram, the atom is ${}^{4}_{2}$He, that is, it has atomic mass four, with two protons. Additionally, it is a stable neutral atom of atomic number two. The two electrons occupy the shell closest to the nucleus. It will be explained below that the electron occupation shell is denoted by $1s^2$. The one indicates the first, innermost shell, and the exponent specifies the number of electrons on this orbit, in this case tw

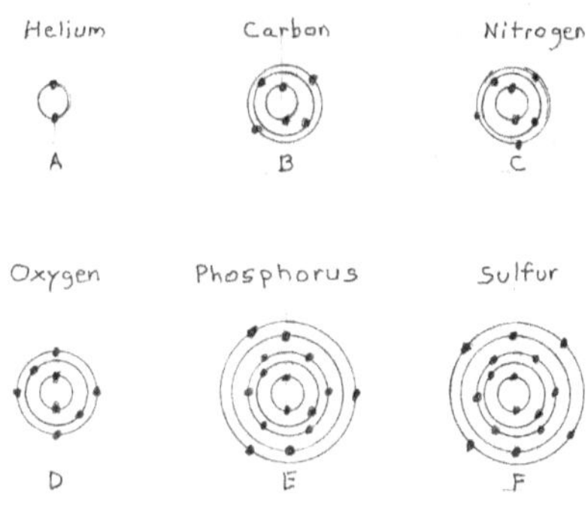

FIGURE 2.2) Electron Formation: (A) Helium; (B) Carbon; (C) Nitrogen; (D) Oxygen; (E) Phosphorous; (F) Sulfur.

Circles within the two dimensional energy diagram are occupied with electrons illustrating electronic shells. It should be mentioned that the location of electrons within an atom are not exact. Actually, they are described in terms of probabilities. This is the Schrodinger interpretation, because these particles are also considered to be waves. The locations of quantum particles when visioned as waves form electron clouds. Electrons do not travel in fixed paths, they travel instead in regions called electron clouds. These regions are most often described as being spherical. The revolution about the nucleus is wavelike, and are three dimensional and referred to as orbitals. Whereas, an orbit is a fixed path, an orbital describes a probabilistic described volume in which electrons are to be found.

Energy levels inside atoms are of uneven levels. However, they are roughly described using the Bohr model. This model explains how electrons can jump orbits only by absorbing or emitting energy. This occurs by an absorption of a photon, or a release of a photon. These are particles of light, and are described in more detail below. Bohr had a probabilistic interpretation, but it is conditional. Namely, that there are probabilities associated with particles, but only if the particles were not observed. The Bohr model indicates that the amount of energy within an orbit is proportional to its size. Electrons revolve around neutrons, and protons, together the latter particles constitute the nucleus.

In general, electrons rotate without emitting or absorbing energy. Energy shells correspond to energy levels having different orbit energy levels. Orbits are labeled K, L, M, and N. The KLMN classification is used in chemistry, indicating energy shells. K is closest to the nucleus, L is second closest, etc. This method will not be used again. Instead a numerical classification is described, using ordered positive integers. One denotes electrons closest to the nucleus, two indicates electrons next closest etc.

Stationary orbits consist of electrons within stable orbits. They do not radiate energy, the energy in the orbit is fixed. Only certain orbits are stable, the ones that are not produce radiation.

Electrons are never stationary within an atom, for otherwise the electron would fall into the nucleus. The farther away the electron is to the nucleus is an indication of a lesser attraction force. The electron potential energy decreases proportional to 1/r, as r gets larger. Here, r is the distance of the electron to the protons within the nucleus.

Photons of energy are emitted when an electron drops to a lower energy level. The energy of the photon equals the difference in the energy levels before and after the jump. A photon is the smallest particle of light. Besides being considered as a particle it could also be viewed as a wave. In any case, it has zero mass, and does not have a charge. The energy within a photon is a function of its frequency when considered as a wave. The higher the frequency, the shorter the wavelength and the higher the energy. Examples of photons include: Visible light; InferRed light, IR; Radio waves; Microwaves; UltraViolet light, UV; X rays; as well as gamma rays, which are emitted as a result of ionizing radiation. As particles, they travel at the speed of light, and are considered to be part of a wave of electromagnetic radiation.

The energy within an atom, as an electron falls closer to the nucleus is classified as having SPDF electrons, Sharp, Principal, Diffuse, Fundamental. This is a method of characterizing spectral lines in alkali metals. More importantly it refers to the shape of sub-orbitals, in accordance with the Pauli exclusion principle. The Pauli exclusion principle specifies that fermions, such as electrons can only exist with no more than one particle within a state. However, two particles can exist, but only with distinct spins. For instance, one with spin up and the other spin down, or clockwise and counter clockwise spin. For SPDF electrons, sub-shells have orbitals which occupy different energy levels. The maximum number allowed in S, is two electrons, in P only six electrons is the maximum. Suborbital D can have ten electrons at most, and in F fourteen electrons can appear as a maximum. This limiting number of electrons can be found using the odd number sequence, in order: 1, 3, 5, 7, Just by multiply by 2 provides the maximum number of electrons per sub-shell.

Orbitals are three dimensional volumes. Within an atom electrons fill orbitals according to a probabilistic pattern. The orbitals are denoted by a positive integer followed by the letters s, p, d, or f. Finally, there is a superscript indicating the number of electrons within the sub shell. Electrons fill lower shells before they fill higher ones. This is called the Aufbau principle or the building up principle. (Scerri, 2013). As a result, the electrons fill up the sub-orbitals from left to right involving the schema:

1s 2s p d 3s p d 4s p d f 5s p d f 6s p d f 7s p d f.

This is called the electron configuration. The representation is extremely important in specifying chemical reactions. Recall that s must fill up first, and can have at most two electrons. Next, p must fill up second and can have six electrons at most. Following is d, with a maximum of ten, and finally, f with fourteen maximum.

The energy configuration is found by adding the superscripts involving sub-orbitals for each principal orbital: 1, 2, 3, 4, 5, 6, 7.

Example 2.1)

All of the following elements are neutral, they have zero charge. In other words, the number of electrons equals the number of protons equals n. The electron configuration of these elements are provided below. The first six elements in the following listing have their electronic configuration illustrated in Figure 2.2. In this diagram principle orbitals, 1, 2, 3, contain suborbital which are closer together than are principle orbitals. All these elements are balanced, therefore, the number of electrons equals the number of protons.

Helium, ${}^{4}_{2}He$: $1s^2$
Carbon, ${}^{12}_{6}C$: $1s^2\ 2s^2\ 2p^2$
Nitrogen, ${}^{14}_{7}N$: $1s^2\ 2s^2\ 2p^3$
Oxygen, ${}^{16}_{8}O$: $1s^2\ 2s^2\ 2p^4$
Phosphorus, ${}^{31}_{15}P$: $1s^2\ 2s^2\ 2p^6\ 3s^2\ 3p^3$
Sulfur, ${}^{32}_{16}S$: $1s^2\ 2s^2\ 2p^6\ 3s^2\ 3p^4$
Calcium, ${}^{40}_{20}Ca$: $1s^2\ 2s^2\ 2p^6\ 3s^2\ 3p^6\ 4s^2$
Iron, ${}^{56}_{26}Fe$: $1s^2\ 2s^2\ 2p^6\ 3s^2\ 3p^6\ 3d^6\ 4s^2$
Lead, ${}^{207}_{82}Pb$: $1s^2\ 2s^2\ 2p^6\ 3s^2\ 3p^6\ 3d^{10}\ 4s^2\ 4p^6\ 4d^{10}\ 4f^{14}\ 5s^2\ 5p^6\ 5d^{10}\ 6s^2\ 6p^2$.

From the electronic configuration the energy configuration is easily found by adding the number of electrons in each major orbital. For instance for Lead, the electrons within principal orbitals are given as:

In 1, there are 2, using, $2s^2$

In 2, there are 8, viewing, $2s^2\ 2p^6$

In 3, there are 18, observing, $3s^2\ 3p^6\ 3d^{10}$

In 4, there are 32, noticing, $4s^2\ 4p^6\ 4d^{10}\ 4f^{14}$

In 5, there are 18, regarding, $5s^2\ 5p^6\ 5d^{10}$

In 6, there are 4, applying, $6s^2\ 6p^2$.

The energy configuration, in this case, can be specified as, 2, 8, 18, 32, 18, 4.

This sums to 82, the number of electrons equaling the number of protons. This shows that lead is a neutral element. #

2.4 Basic Structure of Ions

Atoms which gain or lose electrons are called ions. When an atom loses an electron on its outer shell, the atom becomes positively charged and is called a cation, or just a positively charged ion. A plus sign, (+) indicates a positive charge.

When an atom gains an electron it becomes negatively charged ion, or also called an anion. A minus sign, (-) is indicative of a negatively charged ion. For ions of an atom the electronic configuration is similar to the atom itself. However, it will have more or less electrons on its outermost orbital. An exponent, after the named element, provides the number of excessive, or deprived electrons.

Example 2. 2)

The Ca+ ion is the calcium ion. It arises from the calcium atom by losing one or two electrons from its fourth shell, the valence shell. It is a cation. When a single electron is lost, or gaining one hole, Ca^1+ , or Ca^{1+}, is written. For a two electron loss, or gaining two holes, Ca^2+, or Ca $^{2+}$, will be utilized.

The electronic configuration of $^{40}_{20}Ca$ is illustrated in Example 2.1. There exists 20 protons within the nucleus, indicative of the atomic number. Additionally, this atom is balanced with the same number of electrons. Ions from this element are used for a useful quantum application, namely in trapped ion qubit fabrication. In any case, the electronic configuration for the $Ca^{2}+$ ion is, $1s^2$ $2s^2$ $2p^6$ $3s^2$ $3p^6$. In short, the energy configuration is 2, 8, 8, 0, because $1s^2$ indicates two electrons, $2s^2$ $2p^6$, shows eight electrons and $3s^2$ $3p^6$, again shows 8 electrons. So, this ion is positively charged, because only 18 electrons exist within $Ca^{2}+$. When only one electron is lost in the valence orbit then the ion is $Ca^{1}+$. Additionally, the electron configuration for $Ca^{1}+$, is, $1s^2$ $2s^2$ $2p^6$ $3s^2$ $3p^6$ $4s^1$. The corresponding energy configuration in the latter case is 2, 8, 8, 1.#

Recall that isotopes for an atom are any atoms with the same atomic number, but having less, or equal, or more neutrons than the original atom given in the PTE. Further examples are illustrated next, for ions of atoms and also their isotopes.

Example 2.3)
Cadmium, ${}^{112}_{48}Cd$, is a soft toxic metal, which occurs naturally and is a neutral atom. It is also classified as a heavy metal, and is produced by refining zinc ore. However, the most abundant Cadmium is the isotope ${}^{114}_{48}Cd$. Both isotopes of Cd are stable. For more information see,

(EnvironmentalChemistry.com, 2025). The electronic configuration for both isotopes is:

$$1s^2\ 2s^2\ 2p^6\ 3s^2\ 3p^6\ 3d^{10}\ 4s^2\ 4p^6\ 4d^{10}\ 5s^2.$$

The associated energy configuration for both isotopes is: 2, 8, 18, 18, 2.

Here, there exist two valence electronics in $5s^2$. Interestingly, one or two of these electrons are loosely coupled. If they are attracted to another source, their removal creates positive ions. A single missing electron produces Cd^1+, and when both are missing the result is Cd^2+. In the latter case, the fifth shell is non existent. These lost electrons are employed in forming ionic chemical compounds, and are further described in Section 2.5.

Many isotopes of Cd are radioactive, in particular ${}^{109}_{48}Cd$, which has a half life of 461.4 days. It is one of the isotopes which have a somewhat long life. As such ${}^{109}_{48}Cd$, is not highly radioactive. Moreover, it does not occur naturally. This isotope is created at the Los Alamos National Laboratory. It is a fission byproduct of neutron bombardment using Indium, In. For an in-depth description of fission in the ionizing radiation environment, see (Giardina, 2025).#

Example 2.4)

Selenium, $^{79}_{34}$Se, is a grey metallic looking non metal element. Often, Se is referred to as a metalloid and also it is said to be a mineral. It rarely occurs in an elemental natural state, and is a neutral atom. Its electronic configuration is given as:

$$1s^2\ 2s^2\ 2p^6\ 3s^2\ 3p^6\ 3d^{10}\ 4s^2\ 4p^4.$$

The corresponding energy configuration is: 2, 8, 18, 6. An instance of two ions of Se which are negatively charged are: Se^2-, and Se^1-. This means that stray electrons are attracted to this element and attach themselves to the outer, 4p orbit. These two ions have on the fourth orbital, six and five electrons respectively. These replace the only four elements within Se itself. Accordingly, the electronic configurations ends with $4p^6$, and $4p^5$ in turn, for this fourth sub orbital. The number of electrons are given, for both, in order. For Se^2-, there are 36 and for Se^1

-, there are 35. These ions are also called anions, and the anions with 36 electrons are most prominent. Their importance resulted in renaming these entities as selenide ions.

Illustrations of cations, that is positively charged ions, are for instance, Se losing one electron, Se^{1} +, or losing four electrons Se^{4}+. Both losses are on the fourth orbital.

Numerous isotopes exist using Se. Mentioning several are:

$^{74}_{34}Se$, $^{75}_{34}Se$, $^{76}_{34}Se$, $^{77}_{34}Se$, and $^{80}_{34}Se$. All but the first isotope are radioactive.#

2.5 Molecules, Compounds and Ionic Bonds

A molecule is when two or more elements of the same or different elements combine. Whereas, a compound is when two or more different elements combine. So a compound is a molecule, but not conversely. To combine means that the elements involved form a covalent bound. This means that electrons are shared among the elements forming the bond. A different type of bonding is an ionic bonding. In this case, there is a positive charged substance attracted to a negative charged structure. Ionic bonding is stronger than covalent combining.

Example 2.5)

A molecule of Oxygen is denoted as O2 or O_2. It arises from the atomic interaction of two Oxygen atoms, each Oxygen atom has electronic representation,

$$ {}^{16}_{8}\mathrm{O}: 1s^2\ 2s^2\ 2p^4. $$

Each atom provides four electrons on their outer shell. The result is a diatomic molecule of oxygen gas. The result is very stable since the valence electrons flow between the outer orbitals. The result is not a compound.#

Example 2.6)

Water is a compound, as well as a molecule, because it consists of two distinct elements. Two

Hydrogen, and one Oxygen, H_2O share six electrons on their outermost orbital.#

Example 2.7)

Salt is an ionic bond between Sodium, Na and Chlorine, Cl. To form this ionic bonding, Sodium becomes a positive ion, by losing one electron. Simultaneously, Chlorine becomes a negative ion, by gaining one electron. This is symbolized using the electronic sequence as:

Sodium $^{23}_{11}Na$, $1s^2\ 2s^2\ 2p^6\ 3s^1$—->$1s^2\ 2s^2\ 2p^6$, Na^1+

Chlorine $^{35}_{17}Cl$,$1s^2\ 2s^2\ 2p^6\ 3s^2\ 3p^5$ —-> $1s^2\ 2s^2\ 2p^6\ 3s^2\ 3p^6$, Cl^1-

In this case, Sodium donates an electron to the Chlorine atom. Also, a Sodium cation is formed along with a Chloride anion. Salt is NaCl, and is neither a molecule nor a compound.#

Some bonds between distinct atoms can have both an ionic bonding as well as a covalent molecular type bonding. The next example illustrates this phenomenon. (American Chemical Society, 2025).

Example 2.8)

The bond between Cadmium and Selenium is primarily ionic, however there also exists some weaker covalent bonding. It was seen that, $^{114}_{48}$Cd, has electronic configuration:

$$1s^2\ 2s^2\ 2p^6\ 3s^2\ 3p^6\ 3d^{10}\ 4s^2\ 4p^6\ 4d^{10}\ 5s^2.$$

And the electronic configuration for $^{79}_{34}$Se, is:

$$1s^2\ 2s^2\ 2p^6\ 3s^2\ 3p^6\ 3d^{10}\ 4s^2\ 4p^4.$$

Based on these configurations, notice that Cd can lose two electrons in the fifth orbital. It could lose two electrons in $5s^2$, and become Cd^2+. These two electrons will be acquired by Se, by adding the two electrons to $4p^4$, and creating $4p^6$. Accordingly, eight electrons will appear on its total fourth orbital. This enables the bonding of CdSe. Additional, and more in-depth information can be found in, (Badiello, et al, 1996). #

2.6 Excitons and the Exciton Bohr Radius

Coupling between atoms and molecules occur due to energy transfer involving vibrations, rotations as well as electrical excitations. The decision to bond relies heavily on the energy band gap, and is described next. In the bonding between elements, HOMO is a term used for the largest occupied orbital. It is the Highest Occupied Molecular Orbital. It also designates the ground state, where the energy is least, often referred as the zero-point energy. Most matter always tries to go to the least energy state. Sometimes it is also called the vacuum state. This is the essential concept behind adiabatic computing and quantum annealing. Numerous illustrations of these concepts can be found in (Giardina, 2024). An excited state is any state with energy greater than the ground state. In a molecular orbital, the LUMO is the Lowest Unoccupied Molecular Orbit.

Example 2.9)

Sodium, Na has electronic configuration: $1s^2$ $2s^2$ $2p^6$ $3s^1$. In this atom the electron in the suborbital 3s is in a ground state and could be considered as HOMO. The excited state is 3p. It could be considered the LUMO, since this is the next orbital, and it is not occupied.#

The band gap E_g, is the absolute difference between the energy in the HOMO band and the energy in the LUMO band. For metals, $E_g = 0$, since the two bands overlap. For insulators, $E_g \longrightarrow \infty$, because the bands are far from each other.

Semiconductors have an energy band gap E_g, small enough such that some electronic excitation exists. States on or below HOMO are called the valence band. States on or above LUMO are considered as the conduction band.

Excitation within a semiconductor normally occurs when a photon hits one of the many atoms within the semiconductor. If the energy is greater or equal to E_g, then the photon is absorbed. Concurrently, an electron is emitted and the resulting vacancy is called a hole. A hole is referred to as a positively charged entity of equal magnitude as an electron. The difference in polarity between electrons and holes possibly form electron hole pair bondings, and are called excitons. The exciton Bohr radius, in this case is the most probable distance between the electron and the hole. The number of electrons in the outermost orbit mostly dictate the atom's properties.

The ground state for an atom means that all electrons are in the lowest energy state. When some electron exists at a higher energy level, the atom is said to be in an excited state.

Molecules are comprised as atoms which share electrons forming a covalent bond. In this case, the outermost, the valence electrons are used in filling their outer shell. The electron sharing forms a stable balance between the atoms. Repulsive forces counteract the attractive forces. Usually, a full valence shell results in molecular stability.

As previously mentioned, valence electrons are electrons located on the outermost orbital. These electrons are important for providing chemical reactions.

2.7 Basic Quantum Mechanical Concepts

An overview of quantum mechanics is provided in order to better understand how it is applied to biological systems. Matter and energy in quantum can be thought of as both discrete packets or quanta as well as waves. This duality was shown for photons of light in the very early stages of quantum mechanics. Distinctions were made in this situation on the method of observing these entities. Electrons, as well as several other small particles, also exhibited this duality. As mentioned in previous sections electrons do not have a specific place within an orbit. They exist within a cloud type orbital, thus their exact location is not known. One could only provide a probability associated with its position.

The most basic entity in quantum mechanics is the qubit, also called a quantum bit. This fundamental quantity can be represented as a semiconductor, a photon, an electron, a proton, or many other subatomic entities including an atom itself. There is no mystery in this. However, there does seem to be uncertainty on how quantum bits can exist in a superposition of states. This mystery will be solved by the contents within the following sequence of examples.

Example 2.10)
Consider a modern day classical computer. Here bits zero or one can be considered the two distinct states. These are represented by the absence or presence of electrical signals which encode the states. Instead of using words one, or zero, denote these, respectively as | 1 >, and | 0 >. In the computer, there are only these two states. If we consider the convex combination of these two distinct states, and call it | q >. Then | q > would represent a superposition of | 1 >, and | 0 >. More specifically, let a, and b represent two non negative real numbers, whose sum is one. Then the superposition of | 1 >, and | 0 >, is | q > = a | 1 > + b | 0 >. In general, within the segment [0, 1], on the real line, the value | q >, would appear. It is somewhere in between zero and one.

Of relevance to present day computing, if | q > is observed where both values, a and b are non zero, then this would indicate an error in computation. So the superposition process here is useful in rigorously detecting errors.#

The next example will represent an actual qubit, which is also called a ket, denoted by | q >. This terminology is due to the representation | . >, along with a bra, < . | , together making a bracket, < . | . >. Forgetting this, but again, superposition will be illustrated. In this case it is three dimensional. The extra dimension enables quantum computing to perform deeds that a million modern day computers, connected or not, working in parallel can not perform.

Example 2.11)
As before, suppose that the qubit | q > = a | 1 > + b | 0 >, but this time assume that a, and b are complex number such that | a |^2 + | b |^2 = 1. Then instead of lying in the interval [0, 1], the qubit will appear as a point of a sphere whose radius is one. The sphere is centered in three dimension with the origin as the center of the sphere. This sphere is called the Bloch Sphere, and is illustrated in Figure 2.3.

In this representation it is traditional to denote the qubit I 0 >, as the North Pole. Similarly, I 1 >, is used as the South Pole. Accordingly, in Euclidean three dimensions, I 0 > = (0 0 1), in x, y, z coordinates. Likewise I 1 > = (0 0 -1). Other qubits, I q > = a I 1 > + b I 0 > will alway lie on the surface of the sphere in-between the North and South poles.#

A more in-depth description and illustrations can be found in (Giardina, 2024).

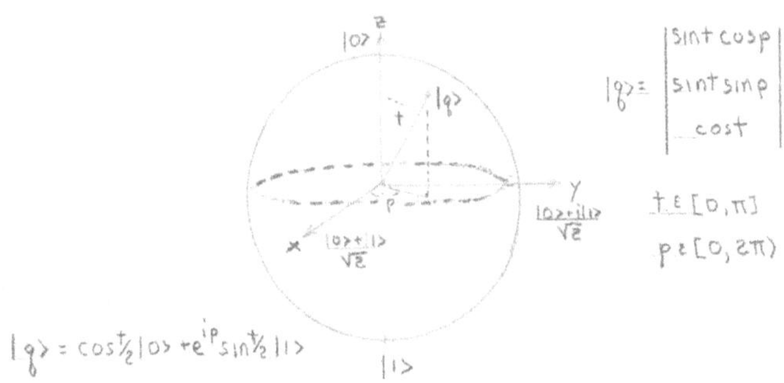

FIGURE 2.3. Bloch Sphere

A question one might have is how are photons, electrons and so on, related to qubits? There are numerous ways. One such is that electrons have a spinning property. When observed from above a counterclockwise spin might be associated with

I 0 >. Accordingly a clockwise spin will indicate I 1 >. Many other properties and features exists for qubits, a large number of these can be found in the reference. Just to mention one of these properties is the coherence property. Of paramount importance is to have long de-coherence time for the qubits. That is, there is the need to stay in a state long enough for completing computation or observation. Refer to the previous illustration of electron states being identified by their spin. In this case, if the angular momentum halts, the qubit becomes de-cohered, and the state cannot be identified. Similar sets of guidelines were employed for semiconductor and other types of qubits.

Almost all of this section, thus far, has been concentrated on the particle aspect of quantum substances. The Schrodinger view of quantum, postulates that the state within a quantum system is completely determined from a wave equation. This is true for all time. Moreover the wave equation is linear and homogeneous. Accordingly if Ψ_1, and Ψ_2 are solutions to this equation, then $\Psi = a\ \Psi_1 + b\ \Psi_2$, is also a solution for any complex valued a, and b. The Schrodinger equation used in dynamics situations is given by:

$$ih\, \partial\Psi(x, t)/\partial t = -h^2/2m\, \partial^2\Psi(x, t)/\partial x\partial x + V(x,t)\, \Psi(x, t).$$

The wave function is Ψ; it is the solution to this equation. In a single dimension of space, and time, Ψ: R x R —-> C, where C is the field of complex numbers. At the very beginning of the wave equation above, the square root of minus denoted by i, is multiplied by h. Here, h is the reduced Planck's constant, it is in the front of the partial derivative of Ψ with respect to time, t above. The particle mass is m, and V(x, t) is the potential energy in the assumed isolated system. When time is fixed and the kinematics becomes of most importance, the time independent Schrodinger equation can be utilized. It is a second order ODE, that is an Ordinary Differential Equation. Moreover, the partial derivative $\partial^2\Psi(x)/\partial x\partial x$, can be replaced by regular second derivative. They are full second degree derivatives, but keeping with physics circles, the partial derivatives will remain. The equation is,

$$h^2/2m\ \partial^2\Psi(x)/\partial x\partial x = V(x)\ \Psi(x).$$

This equation is utilized in both Appendix 2, involving a particle in the box, and in Appendix 3, describing tunneling. The solutions to the equation are employed in Section 3.1, which describes how sizes of the quantum dots effect their color. While the third appendix illustrates solutions that controls the tunneling effect. Solutions are utilized in Section 3.3, which illustrates the tunneling effect in the mitochondria. Tunneling occurs when a particle, for instance an electron, goes thru a substance. In this case a protein. Associated with the tunneling are two probabilities. The probability of an electron penetrating the substance. Along with the probability of it bouncing off, or being reflected. These two probabilities sum to one.

3. QUANTUM DOTS AND QUANTUM TUNNELING

3.1 Nano Particles

Nano technology has existed for a long time. The idea of making useful things in miniature has always been intriguing. An interesting account of the usefulness of miniaturization can be found in (Krug, et al, 2006).

Nano dots are very very small crystals, composed of hundreds or thousands of atoms, and are also called Quantum Dots, QDs. They are classified as semiconductors, and are most commonly created using bonds between Cadmium and Selenium. See Example 2.8, for bonds between these elements. In this case, the QDs are also referred to as Cadmium Selenide nano particles. Their properties depend heavily on their exact size. Size influences different electrical properties, absorption properties and most apparent optical properties, in particular the variety of distinct colors of the QD. Common sizes range from ten nano meters to one, or two nano meters. The color of the quantum dot correspondingly goes from red to orange to yellow to green, and finally to blue, for the smallest in size. The same is true during light absorption.

The result depends on the principle of confinement, analogous to the simplified system containing a quantum particle in the box. See Appendix 2 for a mathematical description of a particle in the box. The result is the consequence of quantum confinement, wherein electrons are restricted to be contained in a small volume. When particles become smaller and closer to the Exciton Bohr Radius, energy bands transgress from continuous values of energy to those that are discrete or quantized levels. A detailed account, and excellent modeling of this phenomena, assumes a three dimensional spherical infinite potential well for the QD. Using the time independent Schrodinger equation employed in the appendix, the energy equation is found. Similarly, the energy is determined in the reference, (Ikeri, et al, 2019). All experimental results agree with the theory of particle confinement.

As previously mentioned, color dependencies are a consequence of the energy of particles in a box, and its dimensions. Referring to the appendix, the energy for this particle is

$$E = (n \pi h)^2/(2 m a^2),$$

where m is the mass, h is a constant, and a is the width of the box. In the last reference a very similar equation holds true for E. There, the process is modeled as a three dimensional confinement. Additionally, Bessel functions are utilized in providing a formula for energy very similar to E, given above. What is of prime importance is that in all cases that the energy increases for smaller values of a. Accordingly, the energy decrease for larger values of a.

Energy is related to the wavelength of the light. Energy E, depends inversely on the wavelength λ. Accordingly, for large values of wavelength, larger box widths, or larger diameters have smaller energies producing red quantum dots. This is very similar to inferred light, it possesses somewhat low energy. The other extreme is blue light, where E is large, and a, and λ are small along with small diameter QD. These nano crystals are tunable in color as a function of their size. An interesting detailed method of producing Cadmium Selenide nano particles is given in (Zhao.chem.uconn.edu, 2021).

Utilizing semiconductor principles, smaller QD dimensions have higher energy difference between conduction and valence band. The result is a blue color. When the QD has larger dimensions the difference between the valence and conduction band is smaller, resulting in a reddish glow. In general, all nanoparticles involving semiconductors behave like QDs and cause fluorescence. The extent of the quantum dot energy band gap depends on its size as well as it composition. Mentioned here is only the CdSe type of QD, but other substances also provide QD structures. Among them are, ZnSe, ZnS, CdS, CdTe, InAn, and InP. Te stands for Tellurium it is, element $^{127}_{52}$Te, and CdTe is called Cadmium telluride. The symbol In stands for Indium, it is $^{115}_{49}$In, also As is the element Arsenic, $^{75}_{33}$As. Additionally InAn is called Indium arsenide. Finally, InP is called Indium phosphide.

3.2 Quantum Dots in Medical Applications

Fluorescence occurs when a high energy photons ,such as white light or UV, excite electrons, causing electron hole pairs. The electron hole pairs subsequently recombine, resulting in less energetic photons. The various energy gaps enable distinct colors to occur. Since the beginning of the century, the use of QD showed an advantage over conventional fluorescent methods and probes for molecular imaging. (Akerman, 2002). QD have numerous advantages over the more traditional fluorescent dyes or proteins. These include:

A longer fluorescence time.

Very small size, and therefore not interfering with the protein function.

Greater brightness levels.

They can take the place of fluorophores due to their color stability; that is, QD are resistant to fading, and photobleaching. The latter term refers to the stability of the molecular structure to resist alteration.

Other benefits are due to the QD's distinct nano sizes. A single high energy source could excite numerous QD in parallel, yielding an array of distinct colors. They are used as optical reporters in human cell imaging. (Walling, et al, 2009). Additionally, they can be tagged with ligands binding to cancer cells and used as cancer markers, as well as for cancer treatment. More generally, a ligand is any atom, ion or molecule which can bind in a reversible manner with a protein. Current research is underway for creating ligands to target cancerous cells with greater specificity, while minimizing off target effects. (iCliniq, 2024)

The down side of QDs are their toxicity. Used as such QDs can cause death. A partial remedy is to coat the QD with an organic matter. The material coating is usually from a long hydrocarbon chain such as oleic acid. However, this technique limits the fluorescence due to the efficiency of absorbed photons.

3.3 Quantum Tunneling Within the Mitochondria

Early on, quantum tunneling was proposed as a mechanism for DNA mutations. (Lowdon, 1966). The publication was said to be the start of the field of quantum biology. This was followed by a text on biology and quantum mechanics by (Davydov, 1979).

Several papers illustrate the effects of quantum tunneling in the mitochondria. In particular, in the aerobic respiratory complex, tunneling is the principal theme in (Hayashi, and Stuchebrukhov, 2011), and (Hagras, et al, 2015). In (Xin, et al, 2019) observation of Quantum Biological Electron Tunneling, QBET is addressed. QBET is observed in the mitochondria cytochrome c. This substance is a heme protein. Heme is usually a ring shaped ion molecule. It is located in the inter membrane area of the mitochondria, and involved in producing ATP as well as apoptosis. See Figure 1.1. In the last reference, optical spectroscopy was employed to capture electronic tunneling in live cells. Real time electron tunneling was also observed during redox dynamics. See Appendix 1, for more information on redox dynamics. This occurred during both cellular apoptosis and necrosis in living cells.

An in-depth description of electron tunneling in the mitochondria is given in (Moser, et al, 2006). In the referenced paper, units of angstroms, are employed. An angstrom is one ten billionth of a meter, and symbolized as .1nm, or 10^{-10}m. Ten angstroms, that is 1nm is the approximate size of a Hydrogen atom. Visible light is between 400nm and 700nm wave lengths. On average, there are thousands of ETC units within the mitochondria. The mitochondria are of length between 2 and 7 micro meters, that is 2μm and 7μm. So, it is no surprise that a single ETC has length about 14 angstroms, or 1.4nm. (Moser, et al, 2006).

In the referenced paper, tunneling of electrons involving cofactor chains of respiratory complexes is investigated. The complexes refer to the results in Section 1.6, involving Aerobic Respiration. Additionally, cofactor chains are sequences of molecules that facilitate electron transfer in the ETC complexes. Referring to the mentioned section these cofactor chains help convert NADH and FADH2, which produce a proton gradient enabling generation of ATP. Cofactors themselves need not be protein molecules, and may act as electron carriers between complexes. Molecules of FeS, more precisely, Iron Sulphur clusters, are instances of a cofactor. A description of tunneling parameters used in the respiratory protein cofactor chains are described next.

Electrons released by NADH oxidation go to Quinone, Q molecule reduces to quinol OH_2, a type of benzene. Subsequently electron from the NADH oxidation drives the proton pumping. Among the most important properties of quinones is their ability to perform redox reactions. In other words quinones can accept or donate electrons readily. However, their production of ROS can alter the redox reaction within a cell. (Bolton, and Dunlap, 2016). Quinones are claimed to be useful in anticancer treatment. (JoN, 2025). The Q binding tunnel within complex I, which is the first protein encounter in the ETC. Complex I, is about 3.5nm long terminating with a FeS cluster.

It is reported in (Page, et al, 1999) that the following formula, involving four parameters is sufficient for providing intraprotein electron tunneling rate estimates within the ETC. The formula is:

$$\log(k_{et}^{exer}) = 13 - (1.2 - .8\rho)(R - 3.6) - 3.1(\Delta G^0 + \lambda)^2 / \lambda.$$

First, only a few of the parameters will be described. The logarithm is a natural log to the base e. Exponential dependence of electron tunneling insulating protein matter is presumed, with distance R in angstroms. A typical packing density is designated by ρ. The packing density describes the denseness of the protein matter, namely how vacuum like or bond like it is. Typical average values suggested within the reference is .76 angstroms, with a deviation of plus or minus .1. Using this value provides a three parameter expression for the tunneling rate:

$$\log(k_{et}^{exer}) = 15 - .6R - 3.1(\Delta G^0 + \lambda)^2 / \lambda.$$

The terms ΔG^0, and λ together provide the activation energy for the tunneling process. However, the parameter λ, specified in electron volts and termed the reorganization energy, is too difficult to measure with precision. Based on this decision, a value of λ = .7 electron volts was chosen. Details are provided in (Moser, et al, 2006). With this assumption, a less accurate two parameter formula for the electron tunneling rate estimate is:

$$\log(k_{et}^{exer}) = 15 - .6R - 3.1(\Delta G^0 + .7)^2 /.7.$$

In the previous reference, it is mentioned that, in biological electron transfer reactions there is little evidence of driving forces which could be measured with accuracy. Accordingly, the value ΔG^0 is set to zero. As a consequence, a very simple affine equation results:

$$\log(k_{et}^{exer}) = 12.8 - .6R.$$

However, in the ETC there is additional knowledge for the energies within the respiratory complexes. Consequently, in the reference, the second and the third from the last equation is applied, thus resulting in more accurate results than using the last equation. Use of these equations provides estimates for the rate of electron tunneling within the respiratory complexes. The method of calculating by using simulations of ETC. In this direction, the two parameter situation, ΔG^0, and R are needed to determine log(k_{et}^{exer}). Tables are provided in (Moser, et al, 2006), along with references illustrating the equilibrium redox midpoint potentials in all four complexes. These charts involve numerous cofactors, for instance in Complex III, the midpoint potential was found for FeS. From these tables more appropriate estimates of ΔG^0 were assigned rather than zero.

The potential energy numbers obtained from the referenced tables provide a starting point for conducting simulations. Applications are made using the dependency on the distance R, in electron transfer protein design. In the previous reference several graphs are provided, illustrating electron tunneling through all the four complexes. Many of these graphs utilize special ring shaped molecules called hemes. Hemes were mentioned earlier.

Generally, a heme can hold, or host an iron molecule. Hemes are employed in transporting or storing electrons as well as carrying oxygen. In the latter case hemes can bind oxygen. Subsequently, they can transport it within an organism. Finally, proteins can cause the hemes to release the oxygen at a proper time. (BD, 2018).

More importantly, hemes facilitate reactions in the ETC. During OSPHOS electrons pass through a sequence of reactions lessoning the energy within each step, eventually, transforming them to H_2O and CO_2. Energy gained in this reaction is stored as ATP.

Returning to the referenced simulations, an instance involving FeS is described within Fig 5A of that paper. This cofactor is illustrated with a rate of 10^5 per second utilizing heme c1. The latter heme transfers electrons from the iron sulfur protein to the heme c. This heme is most efficient in electron transfer from complex III to complex IV. See, (Moser, et al, 2006) for more specifics, and results of tunneling rates for numerous cofactors, and other complexes. Additionally, hemes are also described in this text in Section 4.2. Hemes are used in reference to T cells.

3.4 Other Instances of Tunneling

Before several other applications of tunneling are mentioned, it should be noted that the distance threshold for tunneling is about .3nm to .5nm, that is 3 to 5 angstroms, within a vacuum. (Xin, et al, 2019). Besides the quantum tunneling appearing in the ETC, there are other biological systems thought to involve quantum tunneling. (Dietz, 2025). By bypassing conventional energy barriers, humans can be more efficient and quick in actions via tunneling effects. They also can adapt to different environments under stress or strain. From the reference above, a listing of several quantum tunneling applications are described, a few of these are:

· Photosynthesis - Aids plants and vegetation to convert photon energy into chemical energy. The catalysts for protein, enzymes are employed in electron tunneling transfer.

· DNA Repair and Mutations - Error identification and error correction during replication by RNA. The process is assisted by proton tunneling through hydrogen bonds. However, the proton tunneling could also lead to gene mutations.

· Human Adaptation - Human cells are constantly in a state of change. They adapt to the environment and are often breaking down tissue, and undergoing a repair process. Efficiency and speed of repair are enhanced by quantum tunneling.

· Sensory Performance - Enhancement of human senses and reflexes, and in particular, reaction time. There are theories of olfactory, that is, oder receptors responding to molecules transmitted by electron tunneling. (Brookes, 2017).

4. CANCER AS A METABOLIC DISEASE

4.1 Cell Fermentation, A Cause For Cancer

Having explored the composition and role of the mitochondria in our bodies, we now turn to the thesis espoused by Dr Seyfried, (Seyfried, 2015), (Seyfried, 2025). A summary, of his thesis is that all cancers are the same metabolic disease and that they are caused by dysfunction of the mitochondria. Chronic disruption within the mitochondria results in not being able to produce energy and so it resorts to fermentation to produce energy. Dr Seyfried specified that in the process of converting potential energy into kinetic energy, the mitochondria resorts to fermentation instead of oxygen in this conversion. The essential, and unique fuels needed by the mitochondria for fermentation to occur, are glucose, and the non-essential amino acid, glutamine. Restriction of these two substances would kill the cancer. However, total restriction of glutamine would kill the human patient. Among the reasons for this is that glutamine metabolism products are utilized in producing NADH, and FDH2 in the mitochondria for the ETC process. As such, cells within the body could not get the energy needed in the form of ATP. (Yoo, 2020).

Dr Seyfried basic concept for curing cancer is to minimize glucose intake and induce ketosis. A transition to fatty acids and ketones can then replace glucose. Afterwards, a non-toxic glutamine substitute is given to the patient. Or an anti-glutamine agent is distributed. It is applied in a pulse modulating manner. This medium is provided to the patient for a specified time, and at a dose with a designated frequency. In the reference, (Wang, et al, 2024). it is called a press pulse protocol. Dosage, timing and schedule is individualized. More specifics of Dr Seyfried's procedures are provided below.

Diet and lifestyle have a great impact on controlling the occurrence of cancer. People have control over diet and lifestyle. But they have little influence involving changes in the environment. There is no control over the amount of toxins, such as IR, and nuclear particles that exist in the ground, in our food and in the atmosphere. There is a world wide epidemic of cancer. One half of the current population is predicted to obtain cancer in their life time. In the US alone, 1,700 people a day die of cancer. This equates to 70 US citizens dying per hour. Furthermore, the death rate is going up.

Dr Seyfried's discovery is based on the Warburg effect. The effect posits that a cancerous cell's production of ATP is generated totally by glycolysis, in place of OXPHOS. Glycolysis is the process in which sugar is broken down by cells. See Section 1.6. This is in an enzyme reaction that needs little or no oxygen. It can be harmful because it yields low amounts of kinetic energy. However, it is the only energy source which can be used by red blood cells. See the following references for the Warburg effect. (Warburg, 1956). (Rao, 2016). Warburg was a biochemist, he was awarded the Nobel Prize in 1931. Warburg essentially said 80% of cancers could be reduced by minimizing the use of glucose. Cancerous cells rely on an abundance of glucose. But when pyruvate, is formed it is converted to lactate and not into Acetyl CoA, and therefore does not enter into the Krebs cycle.

The following few paragraphs are edited additional scientific, and more substantive, facts provided by (Seyfried, 2024). Cancer mutations in DNA are caused by mitochondria disfunction. Fermenting glutamine and glucose cause this disfunction. Fermentation is carried out in the absence of oxygen. During this process there is an exchange of electrons between molecules. Contaminants in the atmosphere such as IR do not help matters. Metabolic homeostases is the state of good heath, and is controlled mainly by the mitochondria. Every cancer has disfunction of mitochondria and is due to fermentation. Cancer is cell division out of control because there is mitochondria dysfunction. Mitochondria lose control to halt the fermentation process. Additionally, the more intake of sugar, the faster cancer will grow.

Fermentation produces energy in a slow manner. The fuels, that is, the potential energies, are glutamine and glucose. Glutamine is an amino acid, it is most abundant within the blood cells. It is a non-essential amino acid, that is, it is manufactured by the body. Additionally, it is needed for several reasons including digestion, the cognitive function as well as immune health.

Fatty acids and ketone bodies can be used by heathy cells, but not by cancer cells. Cancer is a symptom of problems in the mitochondria. Glucose has carbon sources and produces lactic acids in a fermentation process. While glutamine contains nitrogen and hydrogen it results in succinic acids in a fermentation process. Together they drive a rapid proliferation of cancer cells.

By using diet and lifestyle changes glucose can be minimized. Dr. Atkinson's diet or Keto diets, can be employed in minimizing carbohydrates. However, the former diet does not restrict the intake of protein. Protein has glutamine within, and too much protein converts into carbohydrates. This occurs mainly when the intake of carbohydrates is low. It is possible to kill cancer cells by removing sugar and controlling glutamine. This can occur with or without an exposure to a small amount of toxins such as chemo or IR. Cancer immunotherapy is now focusing on glutamine. (Wang, et al, 2024).

Cancer cannot be a genetic disease. Cancer cannot survive by intaking ketones or fatty bodies. It cannot survive without glutamine or glucose. Lower glucose elevate ketones. Numerous references suggest using parasitic and DON drugs to manage cancer. (Fan, 2024). DON denotes 6-Diazo-5-Oxo-L-Norleucine, it is a glutamine antagonist. In (Seyfried, 2024), Cancer cells were subjected to twenty different amino acids. This test was performed with and without glucose. Glutamine was the only substance which was found to heavily facilitated the growth of the tumor. It was also found that, without the glucose and without oxygen, ATP was still produced. Succinate acid was the end product of the experiment.

Warburg showed when glucose was introduced in tumors fermentation occurred. Additionally, he showed a high positive correlation between glucose intake and tumor growth. Dr Seyfried showed glutamine is the only other fermentable fuel needed for cancer to survive. Both glutamine and glucose are taken in and used ten to thirty times more in cancer cells than in heathy cells. (Yoo, 2020).

Dr Seyfried claims that there are numerous types of mutations some-six million. Inherited mutations are a secondary risk factor. There is no 100% guarantee of getting cancer when a person has an inherited gene mutation. The ROS causes mutations, which are a result of mitochondria dysfunction. Glycolysis is employed in feeding cancer organisms. The majority of cancers are not exhibited within the DNA. Except for large doses of IR, it takes time to develop cancer. When there is enough radiation, chronic sub lethal cellular injury occurs and cellular disturbance is a result.

Dr Seyfried mentioned numerous interesting facts. For instance, taking a biopsy can spread cancer. Chronic damage to cells cause cancer. Damaging substances include, sunburn, IR, medical radiation, as well as chemo. Random mutations do not occur. Dr. Seyfried showed that cancer cells can even live in cyanide. Additionally, the use of DONs and fenbendazole together induce a greater inhibition of cancer growth. The drug fenbendazole is described in Section 4.4, along with similar substances.

A most useful method for targeting cancer cells utilizing the Warburg effect is PET, Positron Emission Tomography. PET scans aim at sugar when looking for cancer. In this device, a glucose based ionizing radioactive tracer is employed.

The tracer is transmitted through the blood stream. Tumor cells are more than ten times likely utilize sugar than non cancerous cells. PET procedures can locate tumors. Additionally, they can determine if cancer spreads and aid in enabling treatment.

4.2 Methods for Reducing Glucose and Glutamine

Previously mentioned, the natural way to minimize glucose intake is a Keto type diet. Glutamine can also be somewhat controlled by exercise. The paper, (Pedersen, et al, 2020) describes the importance of exercise in this direction. However, utilization of other methods are most often needed. Some referenced glutamine inhibitors or substitutes are specified below.

Glutamine is the most abundant amino acid. It exists in the blood and within muscles. Its purpose is in cell signaling as well as aiding the immune system. Humans cannot stop utilization of glutamine. (Wang, et al, 2024). Disrupting the glutamine intake is described in (Fan, 2024). Illustrated are the different DON type drugs which take the place of glutamine. Glutamine enters the mitochondria and byproducts are used in the Krebs cycle. An important realization is that if glutamine is depleted, another non-essential amino acid can induce glutamine synthesis within the body. It is the amino acid asparagine. Thus inhibiting asparagine would also be beneficial in reducing cancer metabolization. (Wang, et al, 2024).

In a healthy cell, insulin, glucose and oxygen, OxPhos gives off Carbon dioxide, CO_2 and water, H_20. Cancer cells take in glucose and glutamine, they give off lactate, and succinate respectively. Dr Seyfried contends that these two substances essentially enclose the cancer cells. This might prevent anti-cancer drugs from penetrating this barrier. Again, his solution to halt cancer growth is to slow glucose intake, inducing ketosis and periodically utilize a glutamine preventer. In his advice, after a ketogenic diet is attained a modulation technique is introduced. Here, pulse therapy is employed to turn on and turn off the body's production of glutamine. The basic idea is to try to make ketone bodies. Cancer cells cannot use ketones, or fatty acids as a source of potential energy. (Seyfried, et al, 2020).

To manage cancer, a human must only have fatty acids and ketones. Cancer will not survive on these substances. DON drugs are designed to starve cancer cells by substituting DONs for glutamine. These are used when glucose is not present. DONs stop all metabolic pathways which use glutamine respiration. After this, HyperBaric Oxygen Therapy, HBOT is employed when a person is in a state of ketosis. HBOT kills cancer without IR. The principal advice for bringing down the rate of cancer is to make a change of diet and lifestyle.

There exists compounds that have a similar ability to DONS for targeting regulation of glutamine metabolism. Among them is Quercetin. Quercetin is a natural pigment in flavonoid type plants. These include a wide variety of vegetables, fruits and grains. It is an antioxidant, and is known to neutralize free radicals. Quercetin has an inhibiting effect on cancer. Several papers have shown that this natural substance has many different effects against glutamine. For instance, (

Ding, et al, 2024). This article states that Quercetin reduces the intake of glutamine and inhibits gastric cancer, lung cancer and other cancers from growing.

Curcumol. Is said to have a multi-target activity against cancer. It is a natural product and is described in (Wei, et al, 2019).

EGCG, otherwise known as EpiGalloCatechin Gallate, is a compound found in green tea. It is somewhat well known that green tea inhibits glutamine production. This happens because EGCG suppresses the enzyme glutamate dehydrogenase. The enzyme is utilized by cancer cells to absorb glutamine. Other natural substances to inhibit glutamine can be found in, (Eat and Beat Cancer, 2017). In this article, ashwagandha and seeds from fresh peppers are mentioned. The former substance is an evergreen shrub which grows in Asia and Africa. It benefits the immune system.

Vitamin D. This vitamin helps regulate the chances of developing colorectal cancer. However, it does not block cancer, but somewhat suppresses glutamine uptake.

Berberine suppresses glutamine uptake, similar to vitamin D. Berberine works in several places. It has a down regulatory effect by inhibiting growth of liver cancer cells by suppressing glutamine. (Zhang, et al, 2019).

Thymus vulgaris is a natural plant compound type herb used to assault fungus. It is used as an essential oil to fight human triple-negative breast cancer. This substance promotes ROS in tumor cells. Anti-oxidants might be harmful in the prevention of cancer. (Benedetti, et al, 2023). They also can enhance the good effects of chemotherapy on the patient.

Glutamine metabolism occurs in greater percentages in cancerous cells. Consequently, heathy cells receive less glutamine and may suffer from a lack of immunization. An in depth presentation of the effects of minimizing glutamine is given in (Nan, et al, 2025). Of most interest in this reference is the deactivation of T cell growth during a deficiency of glutamine. T cells are part of a human's adaptive immune system. (Cleveland Clinic, 2025). These cells are unique in identifying a specific threat to the body. They employ fission, making additional copies of T cells to counter the threat. These additional T cells are called effector cells. Some T cells become memory cells, remembering the threat. The given reference specifies conditions which can effect T cell performance. The normal number of T cells within a healthy adult is 150 - 1000 cells, along with 500 - 1200 helper cells, per cubic mili-meter. In this document, (Cleveland Clinic, 2025) consequences are provided for too little or too many T cells. Interestingly, the latter might be a sign of cancer.

Since T cells protect various other cells within the body, they have a tendency to also protect cancer cells. This makes cancerous cells less prone to treatment. Fasting mechanisms were discovered to be effective for avoiding or altering this protection Experiments showed that a combination of chemo and 24-hour fasting, using only water, was safe for humans. A 72-hour similar fasting was also safe with a lesser number of side effects. (Gersema, 2016).

In the referenced document, the effectiveness of the diet was attributed to the expulsion of the T regulatory cells which were protecting the cancerous cells. A weakening of the enzyme, heme oxygenase of type HO-1, caused the expulsion. This substance exists within the mitochondria of the T regulatory cell. Heme is a molecular component within hemoglobin. It is ring shaped and contains Iron ions, Fe^{2+}. This ion is a cation, and has two less electrons on its outer orbit than iron, in the PTE. Its principal purpose is binding oxygen in the blood. HO-1; is said to be a stress protein, and an indicator of cellular oxidative stress. It is an important protein used in self regulating redox homeostasis. This protein provides a stable set of electronic, physical, as well as chemical conditions within the redox system, regardless of the external environment. Again, of most importance, is it causes a release of oxidative stress.

Several studies have found evidence that HO-1 increased expression can possibly lead to carcinogenesis. (Waza, et al, 2018). It is reported that T cells at rest utilize OXPHOS to acquire ATP. On the other hand, when these cells are active they resort to glycolysis, which does not involve oxygen.

The mitochondria are drivers of glioblastoma cell behavior. Glioblastoma is a form of highly aggressive brain cancer. A ketogenic diet, high fats and proteins and low carbs reduce glucose levels in blood. Non-fermentable ketone bodies are replacement sources for ATP. They are not used by glioblastoma cells. (Seyfried, et al, 2020).

4.3 Sources Which Inhibit Cancer Growth

This section contains information on several substances that were found to inhibit cancer growth. The theme for this chapter is that cancer is a metabolic disease. There is one cancer - it is mitochondria disfunction. Certain drugs can kill parasites and inhibit cancer growth due to fermentation mechanisms. These drugs are described first, mainly because fermentation is the only means for prolonging cancer development. Once glucose is highly reduced these parasitics alter the use of glutamine. Reduction of both sugar and glutamine is a must in the battle against cancer.

Various other useful treatments to inhibit cancer development are also described. All treatments are identified by underlining the name of the drug, or the method of treatment. Interestingly, several methods employ manipulation of the dynamics involving the mitochondria. Specifically, the fission and fusion processes are activated or de-activated, in order to dismantle cancer development.

Ivermectin

Ivermectin is an anti-parasitic drug, and is shown to have several beneficial anti-tumor effects. These include inhibition of metastasis as well as the promotion of cancer cell death. It also halts tumor stem cell growth and reverses resistance to other cancer fighting drugs, such as chemotherapy drugs. Thus it is instrumental in cancer combination therapy.

Ivermectin is recognized to inhibit PAC1, which is a therapeutic target for certain cancers. PAC1 is known to increase cancer proliferation and to halt apoptosis, however it is a good target for cancer treatment. This substance is a protein kinases and it promotes cancer cell growth and tumor spread. Protein kinases are a large family of enzymes catalyzing protein phosphorylation. These enzymes transfer phosphate molecules from ATP and other high energy molecules to specific amino acids in protein. The transfer is reversible. However, once performed, it alters the diverse functions of proteins as well as their stability.

An in-depth description of Ivermectin and its use as a cancer fighting drug is provided in (Tang, et al, 2021). Numerous types of cancers are specified in this reference, along with results illustrating the effectiveness of this drug. Moreover, illustrations are provided showing bodily pathways for the effectiveness of Ivermectin. Most notably, in this document is a table summarizing the anti-cancer mechanisms when using this drug. There are over a dozen different cancers specified within the table. The schema for this table will be outlined next, along with illustrations.

There exist three columns within the table proper. The headings are: For the first column, the Mechanism by which this drug fights cancer; it specifies inhibiting pathways, as well as attacking stem cells and inhibiting certain proteins; the second column specifies the Cancer Types attacked by the mechanism, these include breast, liver, ovarian, prostate, lung, colorectal, renal, leukemia, as well as melanoma; the final column specifies several References on how these cancers are regulated and specifically, by the mechanisms.

Fenbendazole

Fenbendazole, also known as Mebendazole, is an anti-parasitics and, in particular, it is employed for use as a dewormer. Most importantly is the drug's repurposing. It is an anti-tumor drug. It is used in fighting brain cancers, pancreas, lung, prostate and other cancers. (Guerini, 2019). It is often used when the effectiveness of chemotherapies stop working. This occurs often due to resistance to chemo treatments. In this case, fenbendazole showed great promise. (Hetrick, 2024). This substance was used to treat breast cancer while preserving healthy tissues. It was investigated for the purpose of its redox modulating properties, as well as for mechanisms for inhibiting cancer growth. See Appendix 1, for the redox electron transfer properties.

In the triple negative highly metastatic breast cancer study, redox treatment showed significant inhibiting effects by reducing ROS. This occurred while not effecting the redox locations of normal tissue. (Semkova, et al, 2023). Fenbendazole was also used in colorectal cancer, and it halted cancer growth and also caused cancer cell death. Cell death in this study was attributed to ferroptosis, which is cell death due to an iron overload. (Hetrick, 2024). The latter reference mentions other success stories using fenbendazole, with and without other drugs. In particular, it mentions fenbendazole for use to treat lung cancer.

Melatonin.

Melatonin is a hormone and an antioxidant, It helps synchronize and regulate other hormones. Extra melatonin might promote sleep. The pineal gland is known for producing melatonin. However, along with the adrenal glands they effect skin pigmentation as well as impacting mental stability and sexual growth. It is no surprise that pesticides harm the pineal gland but so also do electro magnetic fields. Synthesized calcium harms the pineal gland, as does fluorine, or fluoride within the water. The latter is also harmful for the bones within the body. These substances decrease the amount of melatonin produced as does age.

High doses of melatonin are prescribed for treating and preventing cancer. This is described in (Shallenberger, 2018). Melatonin is suppressed by all light except for red light. It was observed that there were no side effects even for large doses. For instance, a dose of 60 mg, three or even six times, a day was prescribed in this reference. Interestingly, cancer stopped growing on the subjects when darkness was present. Additionally, it was noted that melatonin inhibits cancer growth and protects ill effects from both chemo and IR. That is, melatonin has oncostalic properties. It is a mitochondrial stimulant. (Mediavilla, et al, 2010). It inhibits metastasis. Melatonin reduces the uptake of glucose, and attenuates its harmful effects on cancerous tumors. Melatonin is both a direct and indirect free radical scavenger. Melatonin protects all human cells from ionized radiation.

Melatonin is made throughout the body, and very often utilized locally. There are different types of the hormone melatonin. The gut produces four hundred times greater melatonin than that produced in the pineal gland. Melatonin acts like an antioxidant; it destroys the ROS. Additionally, it is an anti-inflammatory agent. It is used in cancer prevention and treatment. Melatonin aids in auto immunity as well as in regulating the mitochondria. As previously mentioned, mitochondria produce less energy with age. This often causes death of some mitochondria. Ninety five percent of melatonin is fabricated within the mitochondria.

Blood melatonin can get into the cells, but cell melatonin can't be measured in the blood. The Warburg shift effects cells, making cells prefer glycolysis; it is reported that melatonin can block this effect. (Reiter, et al, 2021). In this case there is an increase in ATP, the production of which is an important antioxidant. It lowers oxidative stress, and reduces free radicals. There are 8000 mitochondria in a neuron, and as much as a billion neurons in the brain. Mitochondria improves the efficiency of the ETC. (Reiter, et al, 2020). In the last referenced paper, it is shown that mitochondria melatonin levels are not related to those coming from the pineal gland. It is also shown that human female eggs and sperm have hundreds of thousands of mitochondria in their cells.

The paper by (Middle, et al, 2025), targets mitochondria ribosomal protein expression, using andrographolide and melatonin for colon cancer treatment. AndroGraPholide, also known as AGP, is a natural anti-inflammatory agent derived from a plant. It is well known for its role in cancer control treatments. The use of both AGP and melatonin together showed the inhibiting of cancer cell survival. Cancer cells can not make melatonin.

The reference notes that enhanced mitochondrial fission in the cancerous colon rectal stem cells promote metabolic changes. These include cancerous proliferation, metastasis, as well as resistance to chemo treatments. This dysfunction impacts signaling pathways as well as energy production. Accordingly, the mitochondria dynamics was targeted in this reference. Using melatonin and AGP reduced mitochondria dysfunction. It altered the fusion and fission processes, leading to a lessening of colon cancer stem cell growth.

Methylene Blue

Methylene Blue, MB, is a synthetic dye. It is an antioxidant, and works similarly to vitamin C. MB was used in the treatment of malaria during WW1. It is an antibacterial agent, and it acts mainly in the central nervous system. MB is well absorbed and indicates where tumors are located. It regurgitates mitochondria by disrupting the energy flow leading to cell death. MB selectively targets cancerous cells, and disregards heathy cells. It works well with IR treatments, and it inhibits cancerous tumor growth by itself, and works even better synergistically. More in-depth descriptions involving MB can be found in (Cancer Center for Healing, 2023).

Ascorbic acid, that is vitamin C, is used along with MB for cancer treatments. Typical oral `dosages of MB that are consumed are, 5, 10, 15, ..., 100 mg. These dosage levels produce very little toxicity. Antioxidants are the most important feature. It increases electron transport as well as creating a greater electron flow. MB modulates functional connectivity in the brain. Additionally, MB is known to perform repairs on the mtDNA. A most important aspect of MB is its eradication of ROS within the mitochondria.

Leflunomide

Leflunomide is an anti-inflammatory and immune moderating drug. It is used mainly for helping with arthritis, but the Mayo Clinic warns against its use when taken orally. (Mayo Clinic, 2025). However, the following development illustrates this drug's usefulness in pancreatic tumors by decreasing the spread of cancer. Leflunomide is utilized along with induced mitochondria dynamical reconfiguration, and is described next.

Mitochondria are dynamic highly moving organelles and are , forming snake type structures. It was noticed that in pancreatic cancer the mitochondria are smaller and are fragmented. (Yu, et al, 2020). Mitochondrial balance is driven by fusion and fission, also called mitochondria dynamics. (Taniguchi, 2024). A balance of fusion and fission occur because of the key effects of Drp1 protein for fission, and Mfn2 protein for fusion.

Drp1 localizes to the outer membrane of the mitochondrion, and strangles or pulls together two sides of the outer membrane. Subsequently, it splits the mitochondria into two. This is the fission process. Drp 1, is Dynamin related protein-1, and is mentioned in (Yu, et al, 2020).

Mfn2 is found on the outer mitochondrial membrane. It works with another protein located in the inner mitochondrial membrane. Together, they pull the two organelles, thereby joining the two together. This is the fusion process. Mfn2 is Mitofusin-2, and is also mentioned in the last reference.

The drug leflunomide was applied to a pancreas cancerous cell. (Yu, 2020). Concurrently, a decrease in the amount of Drp1 molecules was applied, along with an increase in the amount of Mfn2. The results of these applications produced a higher survival rate. This induced fusion promoted mitophagy, which decreased mitochondrial mass, decreased cancer development and decreased OXPHOS. Mitophagy refers to the identification of dysfunctional mitochondria, usually resulting in their removal. This is a concrete example illustrating the fission and fusion processes in the mitochondria, See Figure 1.2, for illustrations of fission and fusion.

Some reports specify that fission occurs to create distinct functional mitochondria. One of the fission byproducts is dedicated to energy creation, while the other would concentrate on other essential cellular functions. The observation was noticed under cellular starvation circumstances. (Thompson, Bates, 2024).

<u>Low Fructose and Low Salt Intake</u>

A low fructose and low salt diet increase the number of mitochondria within the body. This is indicated by white blood cell tests involving the mtDNA. (Hernandez-Rios, 2013). Studies were performed on 36 subjects to see how a low sodium low fructose diet benefits the mitochondria. It was found for those subjects on this diet, that after eight weeks the number of mtDNA increased by 70%. Additionally, damaging oxidative stress was reduced by about 60%. A 23% reduction was found in the amount of uric acid in the tested subjects.

A high intake of fructose can induce cancerous growth. Simultaneously, this intake caused elevated levels of lipid species within the blood stream. Only two lipids, that is, two fatty acids are essential to the body, they are Omega 3, and Omega 6. The mitochondria can synthesize certain lipids. Most other lipids are imported into the mitochondria. The mitochondria are crucial in the storage and oxidation of lipids. Fructose, the most damaging substance, is converted into glucose by the small intestine and with the help of the liver. The result is a lot of ammunition for tumor growth. (Siteman, 2025).

Glutor

Glutor is mentioned in (Reckzeh, 2019). This substance inhibits GLUT1, GLUT2, and GLUT3, and suppresses glucose intake. It is recommended that the individual be in a ketosis state before using glutor. It has an anti-tumor reaction, and induces cell apoptosis.

4.4 Lowering Glucose Naturally in Tumor Suppression

The best way to lower glucose within the cell is to utilize a ketone diet. This can be supplemented by exercise. Regulating and targeting glycolysis involving natural sources is a promising method for cancer treatment. These compounds are extracted from plants, microorganisms, as well as insects, fish and so on. Several quantities are identified herein, and show promise in inhibiting the spread of cancer. Also specified is how these substances effect the aerobic glycolysis process described in Section 1.6. These substances simultaneously regulate cellular metabolism.

Natural sources for inhibiting tumor migration have an advantage over chemotherapeutic methods. They tend to be less costly, more available as well as lower in toxicity, or better yet, lacking toxicity. However, careful use must be instrumented since some substances might be harmful, or the combination of sources can cause harmful reactions. See (Chen. 2016).

An excellent reference for describing about a hundred natural sources targeting glycolysis in cancer is provided in (Zhao, et al, 2022). In this document, diagrams and tables are included which specify the natural products for down regulating, or inhibiting the growth, of cancer. Additionally, with the help of well constructed diagrams, specific benefits are indicated where the natural product interacts within the cytosol. For instance, the table containing about fifty substances that regulate enzymes in the glycolysis process will be described.

This table has schema consisting of seven column headings:

The first column, specifies the Ingredients which names the substances;

The second column, names the enzyme which is Targeted in cancer control;

The third column, specifies the Adjustment Method. This indicates if the substance down regulates the expression of the targeted enzyme for cancer control. It also indicates if it inhibits proliferation of cancer by the use of that ingredient.

The fourth column, indicates the type of Tumor or type of cancer that is targeted.

The fifth column, specifies the Source, that is where the natural ingredient is derived from.

The sixth column, provides the Greek, or Latin name of the generalization for the Category containing the ingredient.

Finally, the last column provides References for each ingredient.

Additional tables are provided in (Zhao, et al, 2022). For instance, a table is provided for regulating glycolysis through signaling pathways in cancer. It has a schema almost identical to the one specified above. Within the rows about fifteen natural substances are listed along with their features. Additionally, there exists a table of ingredients which target AMPK, also called activated protein kinase. This substance influences the metabolism towards increased catabolism. Again this table is provided in the reference with essentially identical schema. It lists about a half dozen ingredients. It should be mentioned that AMPK is also thought to be a cancer suppressor. (Hsu, et al, 2021).

4.5 Glycolysis Based Nano Carrier For Tumor Therapeutics

Besides natural substances to lower the heavy glucose consumption needed by tumors, there exist numerous drugs used for inhibiting the glycolysis procedure. The paper, (Geng, et al, 2023), identifies various drugs employed in nano technology delivery systems. Investigated are nano materials and nano particles which carry the drugs to specific regions. Nano methods will reduce overall toxicity, compared to conventional drug treatment. In the latter case, cancer fighting substances are often not targeted. Isolating the cancers are the first step in the nano particle procedure. Subsequently, navigating nano structures that deposit drugs to these locations are most beneficial in inhibiting glucose intake. Nano dots are also valuable in the isolating, and locating stages for tumors. See Section 3.1, for a description of nano dots.

Similar to previous references for tumor targeting. Two tables are provided illustrating nano drug delivery. This exists in (Geng, et al, 2023). It includes both with and without a combination of key glycolytic enzymes. The basic structure of both tables are similar.

The former table has schema:

The first column, names the Category involving the nano material. It could be a drug carrier, a quantum dot, a dendrimer used in enhancing specific properties of a compound such as reducing toxicity, or some other nano particle.

The second column specifies the Payload, which could be a drug. It could be a protein useful for imaging.

The third column names the Application. These include targeted approaches, gene therapy, imaging, and others.

The fourth column provides Examples of the specific nano device. For instance, the PAMAM could be specified. It is involved in the growth of nano scale pores within cell membranes,

(Dehkordi, et al, 2025). PAMAM is short for PolyAMidoAMine, which is a dendrimer. The latter structure is a many branched super molecule, often spherical in shape.

The fifth column gives Advantages for utilization of nano materials, for instance, long release time, reducing side effects, and the like.

The final column specifies References.

The paper (Geng, et al, 2023) also explains challenges associated with the use of the very small nano materials. For instance, defects within the materials could exist. Some polymer nano particles are subject to toxic degradation. The same is true for monomer aggregation. The latter are individual proteins which might attach, or combine chemically forming other polymer type molecules. In any case, they have a non-stable structure. They often appear in an elongated state. Use of metal nano materials also have the problem of toxicity.

Goals for glycolysis based nano drug delivery systems are listed in (Dehkordi, et al, 2025). These are: To improve efficacy; to reduce side effects of the delivered drug; preventing resistance to the drug. Even though more and more glycolysis nano-based drug delivery systems are employed, the last referenced paper suggests that other oncology therapies should simultaneously be employed. This would reduce the possible drawbacks of a single targeted approach.

Specific nano drug delivery systems target the glucose transporter GLUT. See Section 1.6. Most tumors are oxygen deprived due to their rapid growth, they outgrow the blood supply. This is called tumor hypoxia. Hypoxia is most often found within the central region of a tumor because of the difficulty in obtaining a blood supply in this region. By targeting GLUT with glycolysis based nano drug delivery systems, a reduction of intra cellular glucose occurs. This induces anti tumor cell progression.

Nano drug transport systems are also utilized in conjunction with nano-based Photo Thermal Therapy, PTT. (Huang, et al, 2021). The PTT process reduces tumors by thermal ablation. In this process, nano-based photo agents are employed, which absorb Near Infer-Red, NIR light. In return, energy in the form of heat is created. Local application of NIR light causes the nano photo thermal agent to destroy cancer cell membranes, and prevent cancer spreading.

Normal tissues are less sensitive to heat than cancerous cells. The oxygen deficit in cancerous cells promotes their non resistance to heat. Both organic and inorganic agents are designed to perform PTT on cancerous cells. Gold nano materials are often employed. They are often in the form of rods, or star shaped nano particles. These structures are susceptible to high photo thermal conversion as well as stability. By varying the size, or doping with other elements, control the magnitude of photo thermal energy may be achieved.

Utilization of non organic agents utilized in the PTT process might cause toxicity. Organic agents are often degradable and are more compatible with human tissue. However, they are susceptible to photobleaching. As mentioned in Section 3.2, photobleaching, refers to the stability of the molecular structure to resist alteration. The PTT process can often decrease the size of a tumor, but it cannot completely destroy it. The principle reason for this is that NIR light can only penetrate about 5mm. (Yang et al 2016). PTT can also be applied with agents which are also nano carriers for various cancer fighting drugs.

APPENDIX 1. REDOX And The OXPHOS PROCESS

Redox is the primary step in maintaining the gradient proton potential between the mitochondria inter membrane and the matrix. REDOX is an abbreviation for REDuction OXygen. This process always involves a swapping of atomic particles, often electrons. Assuming the latter particle, one substance gains electrons and another gives up the same number of electrons. The medium giving up electrons becomes a cation, and is said to be oxidized. The other, accepting the electrons becomes an anion, and is said to be reduced. The terminology used here reflects the fact that a reduced substance experiences a reduction in positive charge.

In this case, the substance which lost an electron, that is the cation, is referred to as the reducing agent. It makes the other substance gain an electron, and become reduced. Similarly, the resulting anion, that is the substance with extra electrons, is called the oxidation agent. It makes the other substance release an electron, and become a cation, that is, it is oxidized. Redox electrons are in the donor orbitals, and will be reduced. The reducing agent provides electrons while the oxidizing agent receives electrons, and is said to be reduced. Oxidizing agents are usually in a higher energy state since they can gain an electron and be reduced.

There are Rules governing the methods by which substances become oxidized and simultaneously other material becomes reduced. These rules are not fixed in stone. They involve oxidation numbers involving ions of an atom or a molecule. Ions refer to the excess or lesser number of electrons appearing on atoms composing the molecules or ionic bonds. These rules are employed in determining redox equations.

Basic Rules for Oxidizing and Reducing Agents:

1) Oxidation number, also called oxidation state of a molecule. In a neutral free state is 0

2) Oxidation number of Hydrogen in most compounds is 1, this means it loses an electron, and is oxidized.

3) Oxidation number of a ion of an atom is the charge on the atom

4) Oxidation number of halogens, such as: Florine, F; Chlorine, Cl; Bromine, Br; Iodine, I; Astatine, At; Ununseptium, Uus. Often is -1 in most binary compounds, they are reduced.

5) Oxidation number of Oxygen is -2 in most compounds. It is reduced.

The oxidation number for compounds consisting of Nitrogen, N, Sulfur, S, and other elements do not have specific rules determining the oxidation number. (LibreTxts, 2025).

In redox equations only plus signs can be used. A plus sign indicates that the substances are combined. When an electron is employed it is denoted as e^-. That is, an electron is lost or gained. If more than one electron is employed, for instance k such, then ke^-, is used.

Example A1.1)

A REDOX instance is where a Carbon atom and an Oxygen molecule O_2 are in a combined state when a molecule of carbon dioxide is formed:

$$C + O_2 \text{ --> } CO_2$$

The Carbon atom and the Oxygen molecule to the left each have oxidation state of zero since they are in free state. On the right hand side the molecule CO_2 is neutral. But the oxidation number for Oxygen is -2, using Rule 5). Therefore, the oxidation number for O_2 is -4, since the molecule contains two atoms of Oxygen. According, the oxidation number for Carbon is +4, using conservation laws. Here, Carbon is oxidized since it lost 4 electrons. Additionally, O_2 is reduced since it gained 4 electrons. The method of writing these facts involves to half reaction equations:

$$O_2 + 4e^- \text{ --> } O_2^{4-},$$

$$C \text{ --> } C^{4+} + 4e^-.$$

A note on notation, and ambiguity. The ion molecule O_2^{4-} =

$$(O_2)^{4-} = (O^{2-})_2 = 2(O^{2-}). \#$$

Example A1.2)

Water is formed using a REDOX process:

$$H_2 + O \dashrightarrow H_2O$$

Both entities on the left are free, therefore, they each have oxidation number 0. Since there is one atom of O on the right, it has oxidation number -2. Also, there are two atoms of H on the right, and the therefore, the oxidation number for both together is +2. The sum is 0. Consequently, Hydrogen is oxidized, and it lost an electron. Concurrently, Oxygen is reduced since it gained two electrons. This is better seen by the equations:

$$O + 2e^{-} \dashrightarrow O_1^{2-}$$

$$H_2 \dashrightarrow H_2^{2+} + 2e^{-}.\#$$

Example A1.3)

The ionic bond involving Sodium, Na and Chlorine Cl, as described in Example 2.7), can also be written as a redox equation. This is done with inspection of Rule 4). That is, Cl gains a single electron and is reduced. While Na gives up a single electron in order to balance the total redox equation. Both halves of the equation are:

$$Cl + e^{-} \text{ --> } Cl^{1-},$$

$$Na^{1+} \text{ --> } Na + e^{-}.\#$$

Example A1.4)

An additional REDOX instance is where a Carbon atom and four Hydrogen atoms are combined to make methane, CH_4.

$$C + 4H \text{ --> } CH_4.$$

Using, oxidation number of Hydrogen in most compounds is 1, from Rule 2). This means that H is oxidized and H_4 looses four electrons. The partial redox equations are:

$$C + 4\,e^{-} \text{ --> } C^{4-},$$

$$4\,H \text{ --> } H_4^{4+} + 4\,e^{-}.$$

In this case, Carbon is reduced, it gained four electrons.#

The very beginning of the OXPHOS process is the utilization of NADH and $FADH_2$. These molecules loose electrons to the complexes thereby producing the proton gradient within the mitochondria. See Section 1.6. A basic result is, redox cofactor NADH —-> NAD^+, so NAD^+ is oxidized, it lost two electrons. More specifically, to balance the equation from a physics point of view, a proton, H^+ must be accounted for in this process. Therefore:

$$NAD^+ + 2e^- + H^+ \text{ —-> } NADH.$$

The above equation, specifies that the molecule NAD^+ has a single hole, a missing electron. One electron can fill it, and the second electron can be used in conjunction with the proton H^+, to yield Hydrogen.

Similarly, $FADH_2$ —-> FAD, $FADH_2$ is reduced and FAD is oxidized in this redox process. More specifically:

$$FAD + 2e^- + 2H^+ \text{ —-> } FADH_2.$$

The above equation shows two Hydrogen atoms bonded with FAD on the right, and two electrons and two protons added to FAD on the left. In any case, the equation is balanced, that is the mass on both sides are the same.

As mentioned in Section 1.6, OXPHOS is the primary component within the ETC and the chemiosmosis stage. The latter stage is where ATP is formed to energize the entire cell. The largest contribution to the creation of ATP is the feedback loop containing NADH and FADH2.

Respiratory complex 1 is an electromagnetic engine driving protons within the mitochondria matrix into the inter membrane region. Energy is powered by proticity, that is being a hydrogen bond donor, actually the H^+, hydrogen cation ion donor. The Krebs cycle has input Glucose which goes to Acetyl CoA and enters the cycle. The substance Acetyl CoA spins out CO_2, and 2H, which goes to the perimeter, where numerous H^+, that is protons appear. On the perimeter boundary O_2 is created and also ATP. Metabolism-proticity drives biosynthe. This is the heart of metabolism.

The purpose of the outer mitochondrial membrane is to act as a barrier keeping external structures out. However, the inner membrane allows a proton gradient to occur involving the matrix. The matrix has many more protons than the other side of the inner mitochondrial membrane. . The ATP is created from the proton flow. Within and inside the inner mitochondrial membrane is where all energy actions apply. Proton flow or pumping is created by the ETC. This is performed by complexes I, III and IV involving the proton transfer. NADH, FADH glucose REDOX centers involve electrons to go in discrete steps of quanta.

In ETC the electron acceptor is in the enzyme complex. ETC complexes I, III, and IV provide a mitochondrial pathway moving an electron stream across a redox span of about 1.1V. It mainly goes from NAD^+ and is reduced to NADH. Then it goes to O_2, and finally the oxygen molecule is reduced to H_2O. At the end of ETC, oxygen is found since it has the highest redox potential.

Complex IV, is the final enzyme within the ETC, and does not include ATP synthase. The latter process is performed in the Chemiosmosis step. Complex IV ensures a safe subsequent production of ATP while contributing to the proton ion gradient.

The redox potential provides a voltage level, in volts, V within aqueous solutions comprising the complexes within the mitochondria. This voltage is an indication of the redox action. It determines the extent to which an electron loses or gains electrons within the medium. The redox potential depends upon the species substances Mainly, the potential energy within the valence electrons is of great importance as is the concentration of substances. The temperature is also a factor. Reduction is more prevalent at a higher redox potential.

The inner mitochondria membrane is at a potential of around -.18V. The mitochondria ETC complexes have a redox potential ranging from -.2V to .6V. The complexes I, II, and III leak electrons, causing ROS. This occurs by a reduction of an Oxygen molecule resulting in O_2^{1-}, leading to hydrogen peroxide H_2O_2. An in-depth description of both proton and electron leaks during the ETC process is provided in (Jastroch, et al, 2010).

In cellular respiration, sugar, that is glucose, along with Oxygen molecules produce carbon dioxide along with water as well as energy. The chemical equation for glucose is:

$$C_6H_{12}O_6.$$

The reaction is:

$$C_6H_{12}O_6 + 6O_2 \text{ --> } 6CO_2 + 6H_2O + \text{energy.}$$

energy is ATP. To the left are the atoms, 6 C, 12 H, and 18 O, and to the right the same numbers apply. This is better seen by:

$$C_6H_{12}O_6 + 6O_2 \text{ --> } 6(\ CO_2\ ) + 6(\ H_2O\ ) + \text{energy.}$$

APPENDIX 2. PARTICLE IN THE BOX

The particle in a box experiment is illustrated in Figure A2.1. In this diagram, on the x axis are two perpendicular lines depicting a box structure in between the parallel lines. Three lines are located at y = 0, x = 0, and x = a. Inside the box the value of the potential energy, V(x) = 0, and the particle lives inside these walls. It is assumed that the potential is infinite outside these walls. The wave function is zero outside this box $\Psi = 0$, it will only be non zero for x in (0, a). Since time is not a factor the time independent Schrodinger equation will be utilized. See Section 2.7. It will find the allowed states for a particle to live in the box. Also, it can determine what the probability density function looks like for the particle within the box. Additionally, all allowed energy value levels will be found. The Schrodinger equation is

$$h^2/(2m)\partial^2\Psi/\partial x^2 = -E\Psi,$$

now substitute the value k for the quantity, $(2mE)^{1/2}/h$. As a consequence,

$$\partial^2\Psi/\partial x^2 + k^2\,\Psi = 0.$$

This is a second order differential equation.

The solution to the second order DE is

$$\Psi = A\sin(kx) + B\cos(kx),$$

where k was previously specified. The values A and B must be determined using the boundary conditions, or normalization conditions. Here, $\Psi(a) = 0$, also, $\Psi(0) = 0$. The latter requirement implies that B = 0. Next using the former boundary condition $\Psi(a) = 0$, provides the equation $A\sin(ka) = 0$. If A = 0, a non practical contradictory solution occurs because it must be

that $$\int_0^a |\Psi|^2 = 1.$$

Accordingly, $\sin(ka) = 0$, and so
$ka = n\pi$, for n in $Z^+ = \{1, 2, 3, \ldots\}$. It follows that $k = \pi n/a$. This provides the quantized energy levels. Finally, to find A, using the integral above provides the equation,

$$A^2 \int_0^a \sin(kx)^2 = 1.$$

So, integrating gives $A = (2/a)^{1/2}$, Therefore, the solutions to the particle in the box consists of eigenvectors, or eigenfunctions

$$\Psi_n(x) = (2/a)^{1/2} \sin(n\pi x/a).$$

The corresponding eigen energies are

$$E_n = (n\pi h)^2/(2ma^2).$$

The probability density function for a particle in the box $\rho_n(x)$ =

$$2/a \ \sin^2(n\pi x/a)\ \chi_{[0,a]} = 1/a\ (1-\cos(2n\pi x/a))\ \chi_{[0,a]}.$$

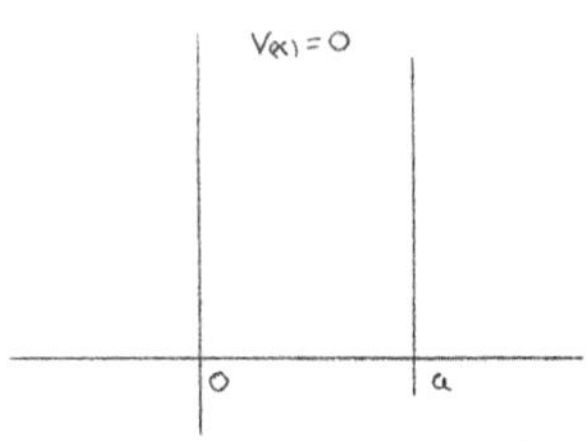

FIGURE A2.1) Particle in a Box

Energies are quantized, and the wave function is zero outside of this box and normalized inside the box. Using the wave function determines the probability density function for a particle in the box. It is ρ_n(x) = 2/a sin^2(nπx/a) $\chi_{[0,a]}$ = 1/a (1 - cos(2nπx/a]) $\chi_{[0,a]}$(x). The distribution function is the accumulative area under the probability density function, accordingly it is given by

$$F(x) = 2/a \int_0^x \sin^2(n\pi t/a)dt\, \chi_{[0,a]}(x) + \chi_{[a,\infty)}(x)$$

=

$$[x/a - 1/(2n\pi) \sin(2n\pi x/a)]\, \chi_{[0,a)}(x) + \chi_{[a,\infty)}(x).$$

The first term in the distribution function is a uniform distribution. However, there is a quantum correction term. The correspondence principle holds in this case, wherein classical predictors hold in quantum situations involving large numbers. Notice that the average value of position 1/a is still obtained. Moreover, the average value of momentum is zero. This can be shown by expressing the wave function,

$$\Psi_n = (2 / a)^{1/2} \sin(n \pi x / a)$$

in terms of exponentials. Use $\omega = n \pi x / a$,

$$\Psi_n = (1 / a)^{1/2} [e^{i\omega} - e^{-i\omega}] / (i).$$

Then intuitively, the quantity $e^{i\omega}$ represents a wave traveling to the right. Similarly, $e^{-i\omega}$ denotes a wave traveling to the left with the same amplitude. The momentum being zero can be understood as the left moving waves canceling the right moving waves. For kinetic energy the average energy is given by:

$$(n \pi h)^2 / (2 m a^2).$$

APPENDIX 3. QUANTUM TUNNELING

Scattering free particle wave solution occurs for the case $E > 0$. The value V is zero everywhere except at the origin. The time independent Schrodinger equation is,

$$-h^2/(2m)d^2\Psi/dx^2 = E\Psi.$$

In this case, since the energy is positive, let $k^2 = 2mE/h^2$, then

$$d^2\Psi/dx^2 = -k^2\Psi.$$

Again there are two separate solutions one to the left of the delta function and one to the right. To the left of the origin, the solution is,

$$\Psi_1(x) = A\,e^{ikx} + B\,e^{-ikx},$$

and to the right of the origin, the solution is

$$\Psi_2(x) = D\,e^{ikx} + F\,e^{-ikx}.$$

Using continuity of the wave function solutions amounts to setting the left hand solution equal to the right hand solutions at the origin. This shows that, A + B = D + F.

The derivative need not be continuous at the origin since there exists a delta function potential acting at that point. It follows that an integration of the Schrodinger equation should be performed. The limits for integration must form a small neighborhood about the origin. Here it goes from minus epsilon to positive epsilon, $|\epsilon| > 0$. Thus, the integral is,

$$\int_{-\epsilon}^{\epsilon} \text{-h}^2/(2m) d^2\Psi/dx^2 dx - \int_{-\epsilon}^{\epsilon} a\delta(x)\,\Psi dx =$$

$$\int_{-\epsilon}^{\epsilon} E\Psi dx.$$

Applying limits gives,

$$\text{-h}^2/(2m) d\Psi/dx\,|_{-\epsilon}^{\epsilon} - a\Psi(0) + E\,\Psi(x)\,|_{-\epsilon}^{\epsilon} =$$

$$\text{-h}^2/(2m) d\Psi/dx\,|_{-\epsilon}^{\epsilon} - a\Psi(0) + 0.$$

The last zero results from the mean value theorem for integrals. Differentiating, and substituting in for the left and right hand solutions shows that ik (D - F) -ik (A - B) = -2ma/h^2 (A + B), where Ψ(0) was arbitrarily chosen to be equal to Ψ_1(0) = A + B. Define a constant β , to compress the solution, where β = ma/(kh^2). So, D - F = A (1 + 2iβ) - B (1 -2iβ).

Now, heuristics can be applied. Say that scattering occurs only from the left. Assume therefore, that a wave Ψ, is transmitted from left to right. Therefore, it can be assumed that the constant A is known. So all solutions will involve A. Also, in this case B can be thought of as being a coefficient for a reflected wave. Since the wave is going from left to right, F should be set to zero because it can not be reflected. However, D can be considered as the coefficient for a tunneled wave. Therefore, the overall solution will be given in terms of A. Solving for B and D, results in B = Iβ/(1-iβ) A, and D = 1/((1-iβ) A.

Figure A3.1, illustrates the original wave, the reflected wave as well as the tunneled wave.

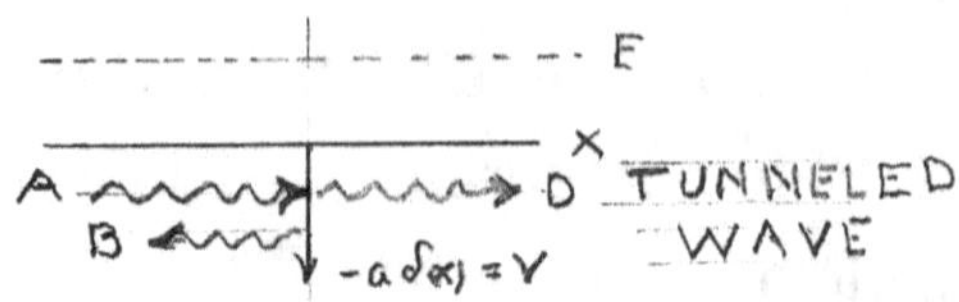

FIGURE A3.1) Tunneling Process

The reflection coefficients are defined using, $R = |B|^2/|A|^2 = \beta^2/(1+\beta^2)$. Similarly the transmission coefficient, that is the tunneling coefficient is $T = |D|^2/|A|^2 \; 1/(1+\beta^2)$. Replacing β by $ma/(kh^2)$ results in $R = 1/(1 + 2h^2E/(ma^2))$ and $T = 1/(1 + ma^2/(2h^2 E))$. Moreover, F + T = 1. To illustrate quantum tunneling, as E —>∞, T —> 1, that is the greater the energy the more likely the particle will tunnel through. On the other hand, the closer the energy is to zero the more likely that the particle will be reflected. In the non-quantum situation, that is classically, these values are equal to T = 1, R = 0 for the potential well. Also these values are T = 0 and R =1 for the potential barrier. However in quantum theory, for the delta function situation they have the same value. That is, if a barrier was used in this problem instead of a quantum well the solutions would be the same. That is,

$$T = 1/(1+\beta^2), \text{ and } R = \beta^2/(1+\beta^2).$$

Again, these quantities sum to one when added together and they are interpreted as being probabilities.

REFERENCES

Ahmad, M., et al, Biochemistry, electronic transport chain, NIH, 2023.

Akerman, M., et al, Nano crystal targeting in vivo, Proc Nat Acad Sc, USA, 2002.

American Chemical Society, Cadmium selenide, 2017.

Apple, S., Ravenous by Otto Warburg, Hypoxia, the prime cause of cancer, 1923.

B D Editors, RNA Polymerase, Biology Dictionary, 2019.

Badiello, et al, Interaction between trace elements: selenium and cadmium, Science Direct, Elsevier, 1996.

Benedetti,S., et al, New insights into the cytotoxic effects of thymus vulgaris oil on human triple-negative breast cancer cell with MDA-MB-231, Elsevier. 2023.

Biology LibreTexts, The oxidation of pyruvate produces Acetyl CoA, 2014.

BD, Heme - definition, structure and function, Biology Dictionary, 2018.

Bolton, J., and Dunlap, T., Formation and biological targets of quinones: cytotoxic versus cytoprotective effects, Chem Res Toxicol, 2016.

Brookes, J., Quantum effects in biology: golden rule in enzymes, olfaction, photosynthesis and magetodetection, Proc Royal Society, 2017.

Cancer Center for Healing, Methylene blue and cancer: exploring the connection, 2023.

Cedikova, M., et al, Mitochondria in white, brown and beige adipocytes, NIH, 2016.

Chelakkot, C., et al, Modulating glycolysis to improve cancer therapy, Review, Int J Mol Sci, 2023.

Chen, D., et al Metabolomic application in toxicity evaluation and toxicological biomarker identification of natural product, Chem Bio, 2016.

Cleveland Clinic, T cells: types and function, 2025.

Creative Proteomics, Pentose phosphate pathway (PPP) in cell growth proliferation and antioxidant defense, 2025.

Davydov, A., Biology and quantum mechanics, in Russian, Kyiv: Naukova Dumka, 1979

Dehkordi, A., et al, Engineering PAMAM dendrimers for optimized drug delivery, Nano Trends, Elsevier, 2025

Dietz, C., Quantum tunneling from cells to systems in high-performance. TriPhasic Training, 2025.

Ding, L., et al, Quercetin induces ferroptosis in gastic cancer cells by targeting SLC1A5 and regulating th ep-Canj2/p-DRP1 and NRF2/GPX Axes, Science Direct, Elsevier. 2024.

Duraj, T., et al, Clinical research framework proposal for ketogenic metabolic therapy in glioblastoma, BMC Medicine 2024.

Eat and Beat Cancer, 2017 Anti-cancer strategies: inhibit glutamine, 2017.

EnvironmentalChemistry.com, Periodic Table of Elements, Element Cadmium, 2025

Fagbohun, O, et al, Role of antioxidant vitamins and other micronutrients on regulation of specific genes and signaling pathways in the prevention and treatment of cancer, NIH, 2023

Fan, Y., et al, Exploiting the Achilles' heel of cancer: disrupting glutamine metabolism for effective cancer treatment, Front Pharmacol, 2024.

Fang, Y., et al, The roel of mitochondrial fusion and fission in immune-mediated inflammatory diseases, Science Direct, Elsevier, 2024.

Guerini, A., et al, Mebendazole as a candidate for drug repurposing in Oncology: an extensive review of current literature, Cancers (Basel), 2019.

Geng. C., et al, Glycolsis-based drug delivery nano systems for use in tumors and application, Bio, Elsevier, 2023.

Gersema, E., Fasting-like diet turns the immune system against cancer, Keck School of Medicine of USC, 2016.

Giardina, C., Many-Sorted Algebras for Deep Learning and Quantum Technology. Elsevier, 2024.

Giardina, C., Probability for Deep Learning Quantum, A Many-Sorted Algebra View, Elsevier, 2025.

Giardina, C., AI Cancer Timebomb, Regency Publishing Co. 2025.

Gugliucci, A, et al, Formation of fructose-mediated advanced glycation end products and their role in metabolic and inflammatory diseases, Adv Nutr, 2017.

Hagras, M., et al, Quantum calculations of electron tunneling in respiratory complex III, J Phs Chem, 2015.

Hayashi, T., Stuchebrukhov, A., Quantum electron. Tunneling in respiratory complex I, J Phs Chem, 2011.

Helmenstine, A., Mitochondria - definition, structure, function, Science Notes, 2024.

Hernadez-Rios, R., et al, Low fructose and low salt diets increase mitochondrial DNA in n blood cells of overweight subjects, Experimental and Clinical Endocrinology and Diabetes, Neurology 81, 2013.

Hetrick, P., Fenbendazole is a veterinary medication introduced in 1974, Heal Navigator, 2024.

Hsu, C., et al, AMPK signaling and its targeting in cancer progression and treatment, Semin Cancer Biol. 2021

Huang, X., et al, Recent strategies for nano-based PTT combined with immunotherapy: from a biomaterial point of view, Theranostics, 2021.

iCliniq, How are Ligands used in anti-cancer therapy, 2024

Ikeri, H., et al, The dependence of confinement energy on size of quantum dots, Int J of S R in physics and applied science, 2019.

Jolly, W., Isotopes of hydrogen, Britannica, 2025.

Jastroch, M., et al, Mitochondria proton and electron leaks, NIH, 2010

Kraft, L., and Lackner, L., Mitochondrial anchors: positioning mitochondria and more, Elsevier, 2018.

Krug, H., et al, Nanotechnology: Assessment and perspectives, Springer-Verlag, 2006.

Lanna, A., and Dustin, M., Mitochondrial fusion fuels T cell memory, Cell Research, Nature, 2016.

Lazaro, E., Scientists find cell-free mitochondria in human blood, Sci News, 2025.

Lee, D, et al, Amino acid and glucose fermentation maintain ATP content in mouse and human malignant glioma cells, Nearo, 2024.

Leija, R., et al, The mitochondrial lactate oxidation complex: endpoint for carbohydrate carbon disposal, Research Article, American Physiological Society, 2017.

Lenzen, S., A fresh view of glycolysis and glucokinase regulation, J Biol Chem, 2014.
LibreTexts, Oxidation Numbers, Chemestry, 2025

Lowdin, P., Quantum genetics and aperiodic solid: some aspects on the biological problems of heredity, mutations, aging, and tumors in view of quantum theory of the DNA molecule, Adv Quantum Chem, 1966.

Mediavilla, et al, Basic mechanisms involved in the anti cancer effects of melatonin, Cur Med Chem, 2010.

Mayo Clinic, Leflunomide, 2025.

Middle, A., et al, Targeting mitochondria ribosomal protein expression using andrographolide and melatonin for colon cancer treatment, Cancer Letters, Elsevier, 2025.

Moore, and Stanitiski, 2014), Chemistry the molecular science, Cengage Learning, 2014.

Morris, G., Berk, M., The many roads to mitochondrial dysfunction in neuroimmune and neuropsychiatric disorders, BMC Med, 2015.

Moser, C., et al, Electron tunneling chains of mitochondria, Science Direct, Elsevier, 2006.

Nan, D., et al, Glutamine and cancer, metabolism, immune microenvironment, and therapeutic targets, Cell Communication and Signaling, 2025.

News Release, Office of Assistant Secretary of Defense (Public Affair), Washington D C, 20301, Oct. 1, 1964.

Nigro, C., et al, Dicarbonyl stress at the crossroads of healthy and unhealthy aging, Cells, 2019.

NRC.gov, Biological effects of radiation, Reactor Concept Manual, 2014.

Page, C., et al, Natural engineering principles of electron tunneling in biological oxidation-reduction, Nature(London) 1999.

Pedersen, K., et al, Exercise-mediated lowering of glutamine availability suppresses tumor growth and attenuates muscle wasting, Science, 2020.

Rao, S., Mitochondrial changes in cancer, National Library of Medicine, 2016.

Reckzeh, E., et al, Inhibition of glucose transporters and synergistically impairs tumor cell growth,Cell Chem Biol, 2019.

Reiter, R., et al, Melatonin in Mitochondria: Migrating clear and present danger, Physiology, Vol 35, 2020.

Reiter, R., et al, Anti-Warburg effect of melatonin: a proposed mechanism to explain its inhibition of multiple diseases, Int J of Molecular Sciences, 2021.

Rong, Z., et al, The mitochondrial response to DNA damage, Frontiers in Cell and Development Biology, 2021.

Russell, J., Melatonin in Mitochondria Mitigating Clear and Present Dangers, Physiology, 2020.

Sabbarwal, S., and Schumacher, P., Mitochondria ROS in cancer: initiators, amplifiers or an Achilles' heal?, Nature Reviews Cancer, 2014.

Sapkota, A., Electron transport chain unveiled: steps, product, diagram, Microbe Notes, 2024.

Sayegh, E., The billion dollar AI gamble: data centers as the new high stakes game, Forbes Newsletter, 2024.

Scerri, E., The trouble with the Aufbau principle, Education in chemistry, vol 50, no.n6. Royal society of chemistry. 2013.

Schuster, et al, Oxidized Linoleic acid metabolites induce liver mitochondrial dysfunction, apoptosis and NLRP3 activation in mice, J Lipid Res. 2018.

Semkova, S., et al, Redox-mediated anti cancer activity of anti parasitic drug fenbendazole in triple negative areas cells, Anticancer Research, 2023.

Seyfried, T., Cancer as a mitochondrial metabolic disease, Frontiers in Cell and Developmental Biology, 2015.

Seyfried, T., et al Considerations of ketogenic metabolic therapy as a complementary or alternative approach for managing breast cancer, Frontiers in Nutrition, 2020.

Seyfried, T., et al, Cancer as a mitochondrial metabolic disease, Frontiers in Cell and Developmental Biology, 2015.

Shallenberger, F., High dose melatonin therapy - an ideal adjuvant anti cancer therapy, IVS Symposium, 2018.

Siteman Cancer Center, Avoiding fructose, 2025.

Su, E., et al, Mitochondria: at the crossroads between mechanobiology and cell metabolism, Pub Med, 2023

Tang, M., et al, Ivermectin, a potential anticancer drug derived from an anti parasitic drug, NIH, Elsevier, 2020.

Taniguchi, C., Mitochondrial fusion exploits a therapeutic vulnerability of pancreatic cancer, JCI Insight, 2024.

Tatomir, J., DNA and RNA Mutations Study.com. 2024.

Thompson, B., Bates, E., Surprise finding reveals mitochondrial energy factories come in two different types, Nature Podcast, 2024.

Vincent, A., Mitochondrial nanotunnels, Trends in Biology, 2017.

Walling, M., et al, Quantom dots for live cel and in vivo imaging, Int J Mol Sci, 2009.

Wang, B., et al, A glutamine tug-of-war between cancer and immune cells: recent advances in unraveling the ongoing battle, Journal of Experimental & Clinical Cancer Research, 2024.

Wang, J., et al, Glucose transporter GLUT1 expression, and clinical outcome in solid tumors: a systematic review and meta-analysis, Review, Oncotarget, 2017.

Wang, R., et al, Identification of new OPA1 cleavage site reveals that short iso forms regulate mitochondria fission. SSPA, 2021.

Wang, X., et al, Asparagine: a key metabolic junction in targeted tumor therapy, Pharmacol Res, 2024.

Warburg, O., On the origin of cancer cells, Science, 24 Feb 1956.

Waza, A., et al, A review on heme oxygnase-1 induction: Is it a necessary evil, Inflamm. Res, 2018.

Wei, W., et al, Curcumol: from plant roots to cancer roots. Int J Biol Sci, 2019.

Xin, H., et al, Quantum biological tunnel junction for electron transfer imaging in live cells, Nature, 2019.

Yang, Q., et al, Rationally designed peptide-conjugated gold/platinum nano system with active tumor-targeting for enhancing tumor , J Control Release, 2019.

Yoo, H., et al, Glutamine reliance in cell metabolism, Exp Mol Med, 2020.

Yu, H., et al, Glutamine relance in cell metabolism, Exp Mol Med, 2020.

Yu, M., et al, Enhanced mitochondrial fusion suppresses pancreatic cancer, J of Clinical Inv, 2020)

Zhang P., et al, Berberine inhibits growth of liver cancer cells by suppressing glutamine uptake, Onco Targets Ther., 2019

zhao.chem.ucon.edu, Synthesis and characterization of cadmium selenide QD, 2021.

Zhao, Y., et al, Natural products targeting glycolysis in cancer, Front Pharmacol, 2022.

ABOUT THE AUTHOR

Dr. Giardina was a professor of mathematics, electrical engineering, and computer science at Fairleigh Dickinson University from 1965 to 1982. From 1982 to 1986, he was a professor at the Stevens Institute of Technology. On behalf of these two universities he headed off campus programs at various industrial and military locations, such as Fort Monmouth, ITT, Bendix, Bell Labs, Bellcore, and Kearfott, all in NJ.From 1986 to 1999, he was a professor at the College of Staten Island, City University of New York.

His industrial career began at Transil Semiconductors, Englewood NJ in 1963. Subsequently he was awarded a Communication Development Training fellowship at Bell Telephone Laboratories, Whippany, NJ, United States where he worked in military defense. He continued in the area of military defense and research in 1968 at Singer Kearfott, Wayne NJ. Later in 1996, he again joined Bell Telephone Laboratories, Whippany, NJ, United States. Finally, in 1998, Dr. Giardina returned to Kearfott, then called BAE Systems as a Senior Member of the Technical Staff.

His research interests include digital signal and image processing, pattern recognition, artificial intelligence, and the constructive theory of functions. Dr. Giardina has authored numerous papers and several books in these areas, including Mathematical Models for Artificial Intelligence and Autonomous Systems, Prentice Hall; Matrix Structure Image Processing, Prentice Hall; Parallel Digital Signal Processing: A Unified Signal Algebra Approach, Regency; Morphological Methods in Image and Signal Processing, Prentice Hall; Image Processing—Continuous to Discrete: Geometric, Transform, and Statistical Methods, Prentice Hall; and A Unified Signal Algebra Approach to Two-Dimensional Parallel Digital Signal Processing, Chapman and Hall/CRC Press. Most recently he authored: Many-Sorted Algebras for Deep Learning and Quantum Technology, Feb 2024, Elsevier; Probability for Deep Learning Quantum, A Many-Sorted Algebra View, Jan 2025, Elsevier; AI Cancer Timebomb, Regency, May 2025.

DEDICATION

To My Betty, My Everything.

ACKNOWLEDGEMENTS

Thanks goes to Ed Cooke for reading the manuscript and making excellent corrections.

Special thanks to Bob Hudson for the great improvements he made in just about all my arguments. While not changing my meaning of concepts, he transformed them into English.

www.ingramcontent.com/pod-product-compliance
Lightning Source LLC
LaVergne TN
LVHW022038200926
848481LV00003B/716

* 9 7 9 8 2 3 0 7 1 5 4 0 5 *